Profiling Linguistic Disability

David Crystal

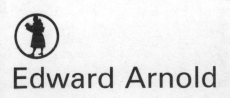

Edward Arnold

© David Crystal 1982

First published 1982 by
Edward Arnold (Publishers) Ltd
41 Bedford Square, London WC1B 3DQ

British Library Cataloguing in Publication Data

Crystal, David
  Profiling linguistic disability.
  1. Language disorders—diagnosis
  2. Speech, Disorders of—Diagnosis
  616.85'5075   RC423

ISBN 0-7131-6354-2

Text set in 10/11pt Times Linotron by Huron Valley Graphics, Ann Arbor, USA. Printed and bound in Great Britain by Richard Clay (The Chaucer Press) Ltd, Bungay, Suffolk.

Contents

Preface

In this book, I have brought together the main techniques which I use in the assessment and remediation of language disability. These techniques have been developed over quite a long period of time. The first was the method of grammatical investigation known as LARSP, which underwent its trials between 1970 and 1975, and was finally published in 1976, under the title of *The grammatical analysis of language disability* (co-authored by my University of Reading colleagues, Paul Fletcher and Michael Garman). During that year, I began to write up the results of research into prosodic development, and the first draft of a prosody profile was constructed shortly after. It has taken several years to give this profile an adequate clinical trial, due mainly to the paucity of patients with prosodic disability in Reading at any one time. In 1978 Paul Fletcher and I produced a first draft of a segmental phonological profile, and this went through some 20 versions before it achieved the final form presented here. There has, in this case, been no shortage of patients with phonological problems on whom to try out the procedure. Finally, the pressing need for a semantic procedure has become more insistent— especially in relation to certain kinds of adult aphasia (where LARSP has proved of limited value) and to the restricted vocabulary ranges of many children. I am not happy with the present form of the semantic profile, but it has proved better than nothing, in attempting to make sense of the complex field of semantic disability. It is therefore presented here, despite its shortcomings, in the hope that it will be of some help to others involved in this area.

The slow process of revision will doubtless affect all of these projects one day. Already, we have benefited from the criticisms made of LARSP, as it has come to be used routinely in various parts of the world. The account of this procedure in the present book, therefore, is as up-to-date as I can make it, being the first full account of the revised (1981) chart. Naturally, I welcome comments concerning the use of the other procedures too, knowing very well that progress will come only as a result of the sharing of ideas about these matters.

I have restricted this book to an expository account of the techniques themselves, along with an illustration of their use from several of the patients who have attended my special assessment clinic at the University of Reading in recent years. The book does not provide a discussion of the theoretical reasoning which led to the development of a clinical linguistic approach, nor of the various theoretical issues which underlie the analysis of phonological, grammatical and semantic disability. I have written of such things elsewhere (*Clinical linguistics,* Vienna and New York: Springer 1981), and there was no point in repetition for its own sake. My compromise has been to add a set of notes at the end of the book, wherein cross-references are made to relevant sections in my other writing, and in the writing of others, which will point interested readers in the direction of appropriate theoretical discussion. By severely limiting my theoretical discussion, I have made this book more into a manual than a monograph—and I hope a useful clinical reference text will be the result. Copies of the various profile charts (A4 size) have been made for routine use, and are available from the author.

There are so many people to thank, for their assistance in this enterprise— not least the anonymous patients whose utterances permeate the book. I could not have begun this work without the support of my technical and speech therapist colleagues in the Department of Linguistic Science, and of those from the Area Health Authority who participate in and support the University clinic. Marion Trim, Chris McConnell, Cathy Evans and Caroline Letts have been the speech therapists most involved; Dr Patricia Scanlon the supervising paediatrician; Wilf Jones our senior technician. Paul Fletcher and Michael Garman have been routinely involved with the developments at all stages, and I have benefited greatly from their advice in relation to the present text. From a financial point of view, I am indebted to the Leverhulme Foundation, who gave me a grant to buy many of the videotapes which are a *sine qua non* of the work. And the University itself has always been most sympathetic to the clinical developments in the Department. As always, staff at Edward Arnold have provided editorial and technical advice and expertise, which have transformed messy text and drawings into works of art: my thanks particularly to Derek Lee for his time and ingenuity. And lastly, my gratitude is due, as ever, to my wife, Hilary, for her understanding and advice while this book was being written.

David Crystal
May 1981

1 Linguistic profiles

1.1 The notion of a linguistic profile, as it has come to be used clinically in recent years, is essentially an application of the everyday concept. One major dictionary lists three relevant senses of the word 'profile':

the outline or contour of the human face, especially viewed from the side;
a verbal, arithmetical, or graphic summary or analysis of the history, status etc. of a process or relationship;
a vivid and concisely written sketch of the life and characteristics of a person.

Elements of each of these senses are involved in constructing linguistic profiles.

1.2 A linguistic profile is a principled description of just those features of a person's (or group's) use of language which will enable him to be identified for a specific purpose. Profiles could be constructed for any area of linguistic inquiry, such as the study of literary style, the investigation of disputed authorship, or the analysis of achievement in foreign-language or mother-tongue learning. The present book is concerned solely with the use of profiles in clinical or remedial contexts.

1.3* 'Clinical or remedial' refers to that class of situations where there is human disability, and where one of the symptoms of the disability is an abnormal use of language. This characterization therefore subsumes all disorders of organic or psychogenic origin insofar as they affect speaking, listening, reading and writing, or the use of alternative forms of communication (symbol systems, signing etc.). Any degree of linguistic abnormality is considered relevant to the study. The main professional groups addressed are thus speech therapists/pathologists, teachers of the deaf, remedial language teachers, and remedial teachers generally (whether in a special or normal school context). The interest of other medical and teaching groups is acknowledged.

1.4 The primary purpose of profile-construction is to enable an accurate assessment of P's disability to be made, sufficient to provide a basis for remedial intervention. The aim is to generate hypotheses concerning the nature of the disability and its remediation, which it is the purpose of

---

*An asterisk following a section number refers the reader to a bibliographical note relating to that section (see pp. 214ff.).

subsequent intervention to confirm or disconfirm. There are thus two main goals:

> (*a*) to identify the linguistic level P has achieved, in relation to the level he should be achieving;
> (*b*) to suggest a remedial path, which will take him from where he is, to where he ought to be.

(*Note:* Throughout this book 'P' refers to patient or pupil, 'T' to teacher or therapist.)

1.5* A linguistic profile is an attempt at a compromise between the opposed demands of routine clinical practice and academic diagnostic research. Ts are currently faced with a savage and frustrating conflict of criteria. On the one hand, there is a growing realization of the highly complex and individual patterns characteristic of linguistic disability, and of the gap between methods of traditional training and the findings of current research. There is a concern to learn as much as possible about the problems facing an individual P, in order to provide him with the best possible teaching, and to safeguard oneself against charges of professional ineptitude. On the other hand, the demands made on T's time, arising out of heavy caseloads/pupil ratios, lack of secretarial help, and other well-known factors precludes the in-depth study which is ideally required as a solid foundation for remedial work. Linguistic profiles provide one method of bridging the gap between the demands of theory and the exigencies of practice.

1.6 Profiles should therefore not be identified or evaluated in terms of the paradigm ways of working, in either the clinical or the academic domains. Specifically, there are three contrasts to be drawn.

1.6.1* A profile is not to be identified with a *test*. Psychological practice has been the predominant influence in clinical testing, whereby a set of standardized questions or tasks is designed, whose aim is to elicit a set of responses; these responses are then interpreted as measures of the character-istics or capabilities of the individual. The value of testing is not in doubt; but there are several factors which limit the significance of test findings, when trying to arrive at an overall understanding of the nature of a linguistic disability.

(*a*) Tests are severely constrained by such clinical factors as time, and the perspicuity of the test materials; there is a concern that tests be short and easy to administer. They therefore inevitably make a radical selection of the possibilities available in the linguistic domain being tested. Articulation tests, for example, typically deal only with consonants, and focus on limited positions in a small range of words. Profiles, by contrast, try to be comprehensive in the linguistic domains they study (see further, 1.9).

(*b*) It is not the purpose of tests to provide a systematic guide to remediation. A pattern of error may be exposed, but before a decision can be made about 'what to teach next', a great deal of further analysis must be undertaken. In particular, some kind of grading must be imposed on the errors, and this related to some kind of learning theory. Profiles, by contrast, try to focus attention on remedial paths in a systematic and theoretically-motivated way (see further, 1.6.2).

(c) Tests provide a score, or set of scores, as a summary of achievement. By contrast, the range of findings encountered in a profile are not collapsed into a single score, but are given a more subjective evaluation (see further, 1.13).

1.6.2 A profile is not to be identified with a set of teaching materials, or the syllabus which may underlie them. Profile analyses suggest paths for remedial intervention, but these paths are seen only as possible ways of proceeding. They do not constitute a fixed set of procedures (as can be found in many language 'programmes'), and they do not add up to a syllabus. Profiles do not *tell* T what to teach next: decisions about intervention are left in T's hands. On the other hand, profiles do give T the evidence needed to make any decision an informed one.

The provision of remedial programmes, capable of being used across a wide range of Ps, is an important long-term goal. It is first necessary to carry out many longitudinal studies of P progress, over different timescales and in response to different methods of intervention. At present, no such longitudinal studies have been completed. As a consequence, we lack objective norms for P progress, and there are few *objective* measures of successful teaching. There is a reluctance to think predictively about P behaviour, and to extrapolate from one P progress to the next. The role of profiles is to initiate this whole process, by providing a systematic account of P behaviour on a particular occasion.

A similar point applies to the provision of materials for teaching linguistic skills. Linguistic profiles are only concerned with the 'what' and the 'why' of language remediation, but as such they give no guidance as to the 'how'. The authors of these profiles, through their clinical experience, have indeed accumulated many ideas about how to teach certain sounds, structures, and so on, and these may emerge in print from time to time (e.g. as part of case studies); but it must be emphasized that such 'hints' are strictly outside profiling procedures as such. Profiles are not 'tips for teachers'. The provision of materials is a matter of T's responsibility, part of T's professional skills. This aspect too needs systematic study (for at present the usefulness of many materials is limited by T's ingenuity, time, experience and resources); but it is not the business of profile analysis to provide it.

1.6.3* A profile is not to be identified with a linguist's description of a language. Because of the greater qualitative sophistication of profiles, compared with traditional descriptive practice, Ts sometimes feel that learning to 'do profiles' is equivalent to 'doing linguistics'. That such is not the case can be seen from some of the characteristics of linguistic analysis which current profiling procedures do not deal with.

(a) Linguists commonly study a specific language as a means to an end—the understanding of the properties of language in general. This concern over linguistic universals is not *immediately* relevant to clinical needs, which (apart from certain exceptions, such as Ps from multilingual backgrounds) are concerned with the teaching of a single language. While the principles governing profile construction are of general relevance, and could be used for

any language, the specific categories represented in a profile have no universal significance.

(b) Linguists are particularly concerned to provide alternative analyses of data, and to develop techniques for evaluating their analyses. A description of a language is not taken as 'given', but seen as the result of analysing the data according to certain criteria. While profiles sometimes include elements from different theoretical frameworks (cf. 3.21), on the whole they do present a single descriptive framework.

*(c)** There is a readiness in linguistics to handle large samples of recorded data, or to carry out complex experiments, to substantiate hypotheses about language structure or use. Linguists are not constrained by time to the same extent as are Ts; nor is there any particular external social constraint forcing a particular selection of data or topics analysed. The only relevant constraints seem to be intellectual and motivational—and the inevitable financial ones (in the shape of resources). The constraints on the construction of profiles place the exercise well outside of normal linguistic procedures. There are, however, several points of contact with the aims of applied linguistics.

(d) Linguists are not concerned to simplify their analyses or descriptive frameworks and notations, other than for purposes connected with the theoretical notion of economy. Profiles, by contrast, are gross simplifications of linguistic descriptions, the justification for which lies solely in their clinical purpose. From a linguistic point of view, profiles are not sophisticated instruments.

1.7 However, insofar as profiles have evolved from the preoccupations of linguists, trying to make good (as they see it) some of the deficiencies in the traditional study of language disability, it is important to emphasise that a linguistic frame of reference is presupposed. Profiles are not introductions to linguistics, and should not be taught as such. Rather, they begin to make sense only *after* a framework of linguistic theory and technique has been assimilated. To use a profile efficiently, one must be in a position to see its strengths and its limitations, the criteria for which it is the business of linguistics to provide.

1.8 In a linguistic profile, certain general principles are taken from linguistic science, and interpreted in the light of the demands of clinical practice. The intended result is a procedure which is capable of being used as a routine clinical tool, on the one hand, and as a research technique, on the other. Ideally, any profile should contain three dimensions: it should provide a comprehensive description of P's data; it should provide a principled grading of the data; and it should show the influences operating on P, as he interacts with T, the clinical setting, the clinical materials and so on. In fact, for a variety of reasons (see further, 1.9.3, 1.10.2), the profiles which have so far been constructed fall short of these ideals. But they are at least a move in the right direction.

1.9* The principle of comprehensiveness insists on an exhaustive analysis of the data of disability, within the limits of the samples of P behaviour which it has been possible to obtain. The motivation for this principle is simply that, in the present state of our knowledge, there is no systematic way of deciding in advance which bits of the data to omit from consideration, without losing information of possible significance for subsequent assessment and remediation. On the other hand, to avoid making a profile procedure too time-consuming and complex, some evaluation of levels of relevance must be made. While all data is potentially relevant, clinical experience tells us that some aspects of the data are likely to be more relevant than others (in the sense of promoting a discriminating assessment or a fruitful remedial path). A convenient compromise, enabling T to both have his linguistic cake and eat it, is the use of the 'Other' category on profile charts—a series of boxes where one can place aspects of the data which may be significant, but which are not deemed worthy of detailed attention in the first instance. The use of 'Unanalysable' is another important time-saving device. Several other compromises will be mentioned in their place (see further, e.g. 2.5.3, 5.6.1).

1.9.1 From a descriptive viewpoint, a profile is a chart containing an organized collection of categories, which represent the structural contrasts available in a language—the various sounds, grammatical patterns, lexical items, and so on. All of the language's contrasts can be assigned to a place on one or other of the charts, but not all are given uniquely identifying labels (as the use of 'Other' indicates, for example). The decision as to how many and what kind of descriptive categories to use is a clinical one—but it is not an easy decision to arrive at. Unfortunately, the present state of our knowledge of linguistic disability does not allow us to arrive at a theoretically 'correct' number of categories which will guarantee maximum usefulness of a profile chart. There are two main reasons for this:

(a) The diagnostic features of many kinds of linguistic disability have not yet been identified, and it is accordingly difficult to know how much detail will effectively anticipate the empirical findings—for example, in the absence of detailed phonological studies of dyspraxia, it is unclear whether a phonological profile chart constructed according to the findings of research done into other syndromes will be as useful as we would like for the study of this particular disability.

(b) The demands made on a profile chart vary greatly, in terms of the kind of clinical purpose T may have in mind—for example, the requirements of a screening procedure are very different from those of a full assessment, but as these two clinical tasks are closely related, it would seem important to be able to devise a procedure compatible with both. It must therefore be expected that first attempts at profiles may be wide of the mark, and that revisions and fresh attempts will be required. The profiles in the present book are all the result of several revisions and long periods of clinical trial; but the author is under no illusion concerning their tentative status.

1.9.2 In arriving at an optimal descriptive categorization on a profile chart, it should be borne in mind that profiles become unrecognizable, ambiguous or confusing if *either* too few distinguishing categories are provided *or* too many. There would be no point in having a grammatical chart which contained, say, five categories. This would be quick to use, but it would be useless: it would fail to discriminate Ps who were different, according to our clinical intuitions, and it would fail to provide a sufficiently specific method of following Ps' progress. On the other hand, there would be no point in having a grammatical chart which contained, say, 500 categories. Apart from the practical improbability of coping with such a procedure, there would be little clinical point: we would be unable to see the wood for the trees, and doubtless the chart would contain many categories that would never be used to discriminate individuals or groups. The principle is plain: every category in a profile chart should be there because of its potential diagnostic value—in the sense that contrasting assessments and remedial paths are likely to make use of such categories. Some categories, or groups of categories, will turn out to be more regularly used than others, and these should have greatest prominence on the design of the chart. But *all* labelled categories must have some demonstrable clinical relevance.

1.9.3 It is this principle which explains why some parts of a profile chart look 'fuller' than others. Not all aspects of language are of equivalent utility, as regards clinical teaching. For example, some prosodic features (such as intonation and rhythm) are more useful than others (cf. 4.2); some grammatical constructions (such as statements and questions) are more routinely used than others (cf. 2.7.2); certain stages of linguistic development are felt to be more criterial than others, with more structures, sounds, etc. being acquired, and thus more places where disability might be manifested. It must also not be forgotten that a profile can only be as detailed as the linguistic research on which it is based—a particular weakness being our lack of knowledge concerning the later stages of language acquisition (after age 5).

1.9.4 A further implication of the principle of comprehensiveness, as clinically interpreted, is that profiles must be seen as permitting varying degrees of approximation to our understanding of linguistic disability. The profiles in the present book are all first-order approximations. Despite the apparent detail and complexity to anyone unaware of the process of linguistic description, they are in fact very general and somewhat simplified statements of the patterns found in a sample. They are to be judged in terms of their usefulness as first approximations; but the approach involved is also capable of being used in an increasingly refined way. The term *micro-profile* has been used to capture this notion. A micro-profile is a closer look at an area of the chart felt to be of particular clinical significance for an individual P, using the same general procedures as were used to construct the chart as a whole. In a grammatical chart, for example, the initial description may have brought to light a poor control of 'Pronoun', and a clinical decision might have been made to work on this category. Before proceeding, however, it may well be useful to do a more detailed analysis of the kinds of pronouns P was using, and the kinds of errors made—and this would involve constructing a micro-profile of this area of the grammar. The same mode of reasoning lies behind a T who decides to work on P's phonology, and who states this aim in terms of 'consonants' → 'plosive consonants' → 'initial plosive consonants' → 'initial voiced plosive consonants' → 'initial voiced plosive consonants as encountered in the following words. . .'. The reasoning which led T to think in this particular direction could presumably be made explicit, but to do so would require some kind of descriptive analysis. It is this which a micro-profile would be able to provide.

1.10* To be clinically relevant, the data obtained in a sample must be *graded* in terms of its degree of approximation to adult norms. It is the process of grading which enables assessments to be made, and suggests remedial paths. Adult norms are used, because they provide not only the obvious comparator in cases of adult disability, but because these norms are the ultimate goals of the child language learning process. But there are several linguistic principles which might be used in order to provide a clinically useful grading in relation to these norms. Simple quantitative measures of increasing length (of a word or a structure) or numbers (of sounds, sound features, vocabulary items etc.) we have on the whole found to be unilluminating. Qualitative measures, specifying the *types* of sound, structure etc. encountered, have been found to be far more helpful. But there are several possible ways in which this information can be graded. For example, we could try to grade the data in terms of its increasing linguistic complexity (as defined by a particular method of analysis), functional relevance (in terms of the range of situations in which language is used), order of acquisition (for the normal child), relationship to psychological variables (attention, memory, perception etc.), and so on. Profiles might be based on any or all of these principles.

1.10.1* The principle which we find most helpful is that based on the order of emergence of linguistic categories—insofar as this has been established in studies of normal language acquisition—supplemented by a statistical statement of relative frequency of use in particular (clinical) samples. We have avoided using absolute measures of linguistic complexity (e.g. number of layers of grammatical structure), on account of the theoretical controversy which has surrounded their use. We have also avoided the use of functional labels (e.g. speech-act categories) in view of the difficulty of giving these notions precise definition. And we have not found most scales of cognitive development sufficiently discriminating to be the basis of a linguistic intervention procedure (though their importance in providing a perspective within which linguistic profiles can be evaluated is not in doubt).

The most illuminating approach, in terms of providing detailed assessments and remedial goals, is acquisitional in character, and this principle is used first and foremost. It is taken as axiomatic that, at a certain level of generality, linguistic categories are acquired by children in the same sequence (though not at the same rate). We respect the potential importance of individual strategies of acquisition, but view these in the context of an invariant order hypothesis. When this principle is inadequate (because research findings are unclear), we fall back on the use of any other formal linguistic principles available (as in the use of a standard phonetic categorization system for the phonological profile in Chapter 2). But in principle, we would like all profiles to have an acquisitional dimension.

1.10.2 Several limitations to the use of acquisitional models need to be borne in mind, if results are to be interpreted correctly. In particular:
  (a) Only certain areas have been sufficiently investigated for a reasonably

detailed developmental sequence to have emerged. The early stages of grammatical development, certain aspects of intonation, early lexical development, and a few segmental phonological processes are capable of providing a clinically useful normative perspective. Most of segmental phonology and semantics, and the later stages of grammar, can provide only very general guidelines.

(b) No claim is made in a profile approach as to *why* an order of emergence is the way it is, nor about the learning strategies children might use in achieving it. The search for a theoretical explanation involves a wide range of psychological, biological, sociological and linguistic variables, which it is the business of developmental psycholinguistics to explicate. By contrast, profiles are elementary descriptive devices, based on a synthesis of the empirical findings of the research literature. Where possible, categories are grouped into discrete stages of development, and associated with chronological age—but this is not always feasible.

1.10.3 The clinical significance of an acquisitional perspective is that it provides a principled way of integrating the tasks of screening, assessment and remedial teaching. By plotting a P sample against an acquisitional scale, an assessment can be made in terms of chronological discrepancy, and abnormality in the number, range and order of emergence of the various linguistic categories recognized on the chart. This might be done extremely selectively (to constitute a kind of screening), or a full assessment might be carried out. Thereafter, the various imbalances represented on the chart can be analysed, with a view to working on particular patterns of difficulty, following the normal acquisitional sequence. For 'language delayed' children, this procedure is perhaps obvious. And while there is no theoretical reason why the other categories of linguistically disabled (both children and adults) *should* follow a normal developmental sequence in remediation, the absence of an alternative principle of comparable cogency motivates our use of it, and the degree of success obtained commends it. There is no 'party line' in any of this: if the acquisitional perspective proves not to be helpful, in a given case, it can be dispensed with, and an alternative remedial path attempted.

1.11 There are several other principles which one tries to take account of in constructing profiles—or at least tries to bear in mind when interpreting them. It is particularly important to keep an accurate record of the sociolinguistic setting in which the interaction takes place—how P is communicating, who he is communicating with, in what kind of situation, for what kind of task, and so on. Sometimes, developmental stages may be postulated, but the relevant (pragmatic) literature is insufficiently detailed or clear to enable a useful clinical framework to be constructed. For the present, it suffices to ensure that the main extralinguistic factors, and any gross patterns of T–P interaction, are noted.

1.11.1* Frequent reference has been made so far to sampling. While the aim is to arrive at a full understanding of P's abilities, it is recognized that, apart from in a few special circumstances, this is not a realistic clinical aim. T's view of P will be restricted to certain therapeutic or pedagogical settings, and teaching must proceed largely on the basis of what can be observed in those settings. In turn, the analysis involved in constructing a profile may constitute only a small part of T's interaction with P. We therefore proceed on the principle that any systematic objective information is better than none, in drawing up a record of P's disability, and that as long as full notes are kept of the sampling situation, it will be possible to take this into account when subsequent comparisons come to be made. In this way, T may use whatever sampling strategy proves feasible (in terms of varying duration, task, topic etc.). Certain sampling norms will be recommended (see further, 2.2, 3.2, 4.5.5), in the interests of accumulating standard samples to aid in the formulation of comparative statements, but these norms are intended for those who wish to use the profiles as a research heuristic. Even for routine clinical purposes, there are certain sample sizes below which it would be unwise to go, but it is not possible to generalize about this in absolute terms ('50 words', '100 sentences', '10 minutes'). Rather, the only realistic advice is: T should continue to sample until a pattern emerges in the data. With some Ps, five minutes may be enough; with others, it may take much more. Whatever decision is made, two practices should be routine:

(*a*) to specify the sample characteristics on the profile chart;
(*b*) to provide an impressionistic note of the representativeness of the sample, in the light of T's own awareness of P (either directly, or using P's parents/relatives as a source of information).

1.11.2* An important implication of this method is that profiles are not statements about P's ability; they are summaries of P's performance, as reflected in his output in response to T stimuli. In isolation, a profile tells us little about how far P is in control of a linguistic category, and gives us no direct information about his production or comprehension abilities. The analyst *infers* this information by interpreting the chart and its accompanying transcript. P's usage may be seen as an indication of P's production ability, or of his comprehension ability, or of something else (e.g. his ability to perceive, or to imitate). To be certain of P's limitations under any of these headings—to make the jump from performance to competence—structured follow-up work would be needed.

1.12 There are six stages in profiling procedure:

(*i*) a sample of P data is obtained;
(*ii*) the sample is transcribed;
(*iii*) the transcription is analysed;
(*iv*) the analysis is profiled on a summary chart;
(*v*) the pattern on the profile chart is assessed;
(*vi*) the profile pattern is given an interpretation in remedial terms.

The techniques involved in each of these stages are illustrated in Chapters 2 5.

1.12.1 The crucial role of the transcriptional record (stage (*ii*)) should be noted. A summary of P's usage on a chart in categorical form, with accompanying statistics, is an important first step, in that it enables previously-unnoticed gross patterns to emerge. The awareness of these patterns may be enough for an initial assessment or statement of remedial goals. But often the profile pattern is unexpected, ambiguous or contradictory. For example, imbalances in grammatical or phonological profiles may be due to an abnormal use of certain lexical items, e.g. frequent use of the item *panda* would produce a high total for a medial [nd] cluster, when there might be little evidence of other clusters in the data; a high total for *Adjective + Noun* would seem less significant if the bulk of the adjectives turned out to be the item *red*. It is impossible to get all interesting information onto a profile chart—hence the importance of having a transcription available to refer to, in order to check the validity of one's findings, and to suggest explanations of curious patterns.

1.12.2 The reliability of one's transcription is thus a point of some importance. It is impracticable to keep referring back to the audio-/videotape record—nor should it be necessary, if an adequate transcription has been made. The data transcription, whether phonological, grammatical or semantic, is likely to be the most time-consuming part of the whole profile exercise, but it must not be skimped—the validity of a profile depends entirely upon its accuracy. A small amount of data well transcribed is far more valuable than a casual transcription of a large corpus. It should also be noted that transcription involves more than writing down what P (and T) has said: it means providing sufficient contextualization to enable T to see afterwards what P meant. It is unlikely that this can be done efficiently other than by the profile analyst; moreover, the exercise of trying to work out for oneself what P was saying and intending can itself be an extremely illuminating guide to P's disability.

1.12.3 There are 3 main features of the kinds of transcription we have used for speech samples:

(i) Each sentence that T or P uses is placed on a separate line. This is to provide an immediate impression of the nature of the interaction, and to facilitate the sentence-counting procedure (see further, 2.17). It also forces the analyst to face up to the fundamental question of how far P is able to organize his utterance into sentence units.

(ii) Each page of transcription has a right-hand margin, in which is placed any extralinguistic information necessary to interpret the transcription (e.g. facts about what P is doing, or what materials are being used, which cannot be gleaned from the speech of the participants). This margin can also be used for information about any speech characteristics which the basic transcription does not provide.

(iii) A simplified prosodic transcription is made of both T and P speech, the main features of which are given below. The way P organizes his speech prosodically is the main clue to the organisation of his grammar, and a full account of grammatical disability cannot be obtained without this dimension. It is appreciated that many Ts have had little or no training in the prosody of speech, but this does not alter the facts: many fundamental questions concerning the identity of sentence-units and their constituents, and the way

sentences function, cannot be answered without prosodic information. The use of everyday punctuation gives a hint of the prosodic organization of speech, but is far too incomplete and ambiguous to be reliable.

1.12.4 The prosodic features used are explained in Chapter 4. Five main features are involved:

(i) Tone-units are marked by slant lines (see further, 4.3.1), e.g.
the man is walking/.
(ii) The direction of the nuclear tone is marked by an accent, whether falling (ˋ), rising (ˊ), level (ˉ) or (occasionally) falling-rising (ˇ) or rising-falling (ˆ) (see further, 4.3.3), e.g.
màn/   státion/
The accent is always placed above the vowel of (the stressed syllable of) a word.
(iii) The nuclear tone is placed on the word which is maximally prominent in the tone-unit, e.g.
the 'man is wàlking/   the màn is 'walking/
(iv) Other prominent syllables in the tone-unit are indicated by a stress-mark (').
(v) Degrees of pause length are indicated by a four-term system: brief (.); unit (equivalent to a pulse of a speaker's rhythm) (–); double (––); and treble (–––). Longer pauses are subsumed under treble.

Other features of the transcription are:

(i) uninterpretable speech is placed in ( ); it may be phonetically transcribed, or its pattern indicated more vaguely, e.g. *(2 syllables)*. A stretch of orthographic transcription enclosed in parenthesis indicates that the analyst is unsure as to what is on the tape, e.g. *he said (that he) was coming/*. A question-mark before a word indicates a doubt about the transcriptional accuracy of that word, e.g. *holding ?a cat/*.
(ii) Nonlinguistic vocal information is written into the transcript at the appropriate point, e.g. *laughs*.
(iii) If the participants overlap in their speech, the point of overlap is marked with asterisks, e.g.

T   I think he is *walking/
P   *he walking/

(iv) A brief or incomplete utterance which does not interrupt the speaker's flow is indicated at the point it occurs using double parentheses, e.g.
him is is ((m)) walking/
(v) Capital letters are not needed at the beginnings of sentences, but they are kept for ease of reading in the case of proper names, abbreviations, and the pronoun *I*.

A typical piece of transcription is as follows:

T   Jŏhn/
      lìsten/ ––   *holds up blue and red pencils*
      'show me the blùe 'pencil/ –
P   thère/   *points to blue pencil*

T	'that's rîght/	
	'good bòy/	
	'now *show	
P	*'that blùe 'one/	
T	yès/	
	it ìs/ .	
	'now lîsten/ –	
	'show me the rèd 'pencil/	
P	– – –	*points to red pencil*
T	'very gòod/ – –	*puts red pencil in a box*
	nòw 'tell me/ .	
	'where's the rèd 'pencil 'gone/	
P	in thère/ – –	*points to box*
T	whére/	
P	'in . *(1 syll)* thàt/	

Orthographic transcription suffices for the analysis of prosodic, grammatical and semantic disability. For a segmental phonological profile, however, a phonetic transcription of some type is required (see further, Chapter 3).

1.13 It can be seen from the above that the essential strength of a profile procedure is the way in which it makes T look at P's language in a systematic and detailed way, and organizes the data in such a way that clinically relevant patterns emerge. A wide range of patterns will be seen as T scrutinizes a profile chart, and each will be evaluated for its remedial significance. No attempt is made to summarize the data into a single score. From the viewpoint of linguistics, these aims are not very ambitious; but from the clinical viewpoint, they constitute a major advance. It must be recalled that few published descriptions of individual Ps exist—and I know of no description of any P which provides a 'macroprofile', in which all the factors addressed in this book are incorporated, and the interactions between them probed.

1.13.1 At the level of 'first approximation', four main profiling procedures are outlined and illustrated in Chapters 2–5—one for each of the 'traditional' linguistic levels of grammar and semantics, and two for phonology. They are used, where appropriate, for Ps manifesting disability in these areas.

(a) The grammatical procedure known as LARSP is reviewed in Chapter 2, in its 1981 revision. In retrospect, the title now seems over-ambitious; instead of '*Language* Assessment, Remediation and Screening Procedure', it could more usefully be labelled 'Grammatical Assessment. . .'—if the acronym GRARSP stood any chance of being accepted!

(b) The segmental phonological procedure described in Chapter 2 incorporates an (optional) separate quantitative summary: the procedure is referred to as PROPH ('*Pro*file in *Ph*onology').

(c) The nonsegmental phonological procedure described in Chapter 3 is primarily an analysis of prosodic features, especially intonation: it is referred to as PROP ('*Pro*sody *P*rofile').

(d) The semantic procedure described in Chapter 4 incorporates both

lexical and grammatical dimensions: it is referred to as PRISM ('*Profile In Semantics*').

1.13.2 The extent to which a statistical dimension can or should be formally incorporated into these procedures is left open by this book, but it is a matter which warrants close attention. T makes impressionistic frequency judgements as a matter of course, in using profiles, and it would be helpful if these could be made precise. However, in the absence of published frequency norms for most of the linguistic categories and constructions in the different varieties of child or adult spoken English, it is difficult to make our normative intuitions explicit, and thus to provide a formal procedure for evaluating the divergence of clinical samples from these norms. The best we can do is identify certain general statistical characteristics of the clinical samples, in such a way that imbalance in the use of categories can be highlighted. In the case of PROPH, an illustration of such a summarizing procedure is presented. Doubtless as computational processing of clinical data becomes more practicable, such summaries will become more routine, for all aspects of the work, and interesting statistical correlations come to be demonstrated. The use of linguistic profiles is in its infancy.

2 LARSP

2.1* The approach to grammatical disability known as LARSP (Language Assessment, Remediation and Screening Procedure) is summarized in the form of a single-page profile chart, on which the various patterns of grammatical strength and weakness in a clinical sample can be plotted. The profile chart contains several kinds of information, organized in terms of three main dimensions:

    (a) the main types of organization in sentence structure and function are represented under various headings laid out horizontally on the chart;
    (b) the main stages of grammatical acquisition are laid out vertically on the chart, beneath the thick black line;
    (c) the main patterns of grammatical interaction between T and P are summarized above the thick black line, in Sections B, C and D.

In addition, the bottom line of the chart contains certain kinds of summarizing information, and Section A is included primarily as a time-saving device in using the procedure.

These kinds of information may be summarized in the outline chart on p. 15.

2.2* For a full assessment, it is recommended that a sample of approximately 30 minutes' duration be obtained of an unstructured T/P interaction, using whatever stimuli are felt likely to facilitate a free conversation (e.g. toys, pictures, magazines, questions about pastimes). In practice, it is recognized that it is often impossible to obtain such a sample, and that various kinds of structuring may need to be introduced into the situation. All relevant variables (e.g. type of materials used, number of participants, character of any formal stimuli) should be noted on the top of the chart. Likewise, if a shorter (or longer) sample has been taken, this too should be indicated at the top of the chart.

Whatever the size and type of sample, T should try to obtain P responses relating to two types of stimuli: *(i)* stimuli relating to the immediate environment of their interaction (e.g. questions about the room they are in, or about the toys or pictures being used); *(ii)* stimuli relating to objects, events, etc. *not* visible to T or P (e.g. recent events in P's life, what is about to happen to P). This is to ensure that a reasonable opportunity is given for P to use a wide range of structures, relating to both types of situation—different tense forms, for example. A similar distinction should be borne in mind if written or signed samples are being used as input to a LARSP analysis.

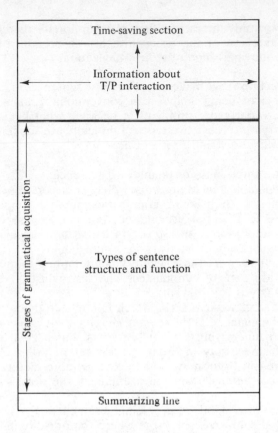

2.3* It is important to make as full a transcription as possible of any spoken or signed sample. P's speech is usually too complex to allow a grammatical analysis to be made 'off the cuff'; and in those cases where P is saying little or nothing, the need to look carefully at the nature of T's stimuli and reactions is paramount. A certain amount of time may be saved by not transcribing parts of T's speech which are plainly irrelevant to P's response pattern, and sometimes one need not transcribe T's intonation and pauses (unless the P analysis is likely to be affected by considerations related to the prosodic organisation of T's speech—as is the case with problems of short-term memory and attention, for example). But in general, one must expect to have to spend time on obtaining an adequate transcription as the basis for a grammatical analysis (cf. 1.12.2).

2.4 A grammatical and interactional analysis is made of the sentences found in the transcribed sample, and the information transferred to the profile chart. There are several possible ways of carrying out these stages of the investigation. Some analysts prefer to carry out the whole of the grammatical analysis before beginning the process of marking up the profile chart; others prefer to profile each sentence as it is analysed. Some analysts prefer to profile the acquisitional stages before the interactional sections (B, C and D);

others prefer to study interaction first. What follows is therefore not a guide as to the routine use of the procedure, but an account of the categories recognised on the chart, and of their organization.

2.5* Under Section A we make a note of those sentences in the sample which are not capable of being analysed in conventional grammatical terms, or where there are particular problems in deciding what kind of grammatical analysis to carry out. These two types of difficulty are summarized under the headings of *Unanalysed* and *Problematic*.

2.5.1 There are three kinds of unanalysed sentence:

(i) Unintelligible sentences are those where some or all of the language is sufficiently unclear to make a grammatical analysis impossible. This is commonly due to P's poor articulation, but it may also be due to poor recording, external noises, and so on. In the written language, the relevant problems will include poor handwriting, smudging etc.

(ii) Symbolic noises are those where P is attempting to mimic noises from the real world, e.g. of ambulances, horses, whistles. In such cases, grammatical analysis is irrelevant.

(iii) Deviant sentences are those which fall outside the normal patterns of child or adult language, e.g. *the cat a kicked, there my is washing man*. There may be pattern underlying deviant sentences, but a great deal of analytic work would be necessary in order to discover it. All such sentences are therefore placed in Section A, and looked at more closely only if a clear pattern does not emerge from the profiling of the non-deviant sentences.

2.5.2 There are three kinds of problematic sentences:

(i) Incomplete sentences are those where the prosody indicates that (for whatever reason) a sentence remains unfinished, e.g. *the 'man is . . .* The initial part of the sentence may be quite clear, but the incompleteness makes it impossible to assign the utterance to a particular part of the chart. Lack of graphic clues sometimes indicates an incomplete sentence in written language.

(ii) Ambiguous sentences are those where, having taken context into account, it is unclear what grammatical analysis to assign to a sentence. P, pointing at a picture, might say *măn/ – càr/*, for example—two separate tone-units with a short pause in between: it would be unclear whether this was to be taken as one (two-word) sentence, or two (single-word) sentences. If a decision cannot be made, the Ambiguous category should be used.

(iii) Stereotyped sentences are those where all or part of a construction has been learned as a single unit, e.g. *how do you do?, least said, soonest mended*. Such sentences do not permit the application of the normal grammatical rules of the language. Stereotyped speech or writing is a common feature of linguistic disability, often just part of a sentence being affected, e.g. if P tended to start a series of sentences in the same way. Abnormal patterns of stereotyped phrasing may be encountered—one P used the phrase *me colour bus,* without meaning and regardless of context. All such sentences are placed in Section A, and looked at more closely only if a clear pattern does not emerge from the profiling of the non-stereotyped sentences.

2.5.3 While the main purpose of Section A is to save time—enabling T to note the occurrence of an awkward sentence on the chart without having to spend time attempting to analyse it straight away—the information it contains can often be helpful, in carrying out an assessment. For example, the proportion of Unintelligible sentences in a sample can be an interesting index of the nature of the problem. Deviant sentences can sometimes throw light on the weakest points in P's grammatical ability. Incomplete sentences may tell us something about P's limitations in memory, attention or linguistic processing. It should be emphasised that assigning a sentence to Section A is a temporary measure. Its purpose is to enable T to get on with the analysis of the clear sentences in the sample—usually the majority. But it is always possible to look again at the Section A sentences at a later stage of investigation.

Section A is laid out as follows:

A	Unanalysed			Problematic		
	1 Unintelligible	2 Symbolic Noise	3 Deviant	1 Incom- plete	2 Ambig- uous	3 Stereo- types

2.6* The acquisitional part of the chart is located below the thick black line. Seven stages in the learning of sentence structure are recognized. Each stage is identified by the main grammatical processes which seem to be operating within it, and is given an approximate chronological age-range for its acquisition by normal children. It should be emphasised that these age-ranges are averages, based on a synthesis of research findings in normal language acquisition. Individual differences in the rate of acquisition are therefore to be expected. But the order of emergence of the grammatical patterns is held to be constant.

2.7* Stage I runs from about 9 months to about 1½ years (0;9–1;6). At this stage, sentences are restricted to single words or word-like units. Two types of sentence are recognized: Minor and Major. Major sentences are those whose elements are able to combine with other elements according to the language's grammatical rules, to produce an indefinitely large set of sentences. Minor sentences, by contrast, do not permit the application of these rules, and do not readily allow an analysis into structural types. Major sentence patterns, in other words, are productive; minor sentences are not. Minor sentences are nonetheless very frequent in clinical conversation.

2.7.1 Four headings are devoted to the classification of Minor sentence at Stage I:

(i) Responses, such as *yes, no, mhm;*
(ii) Vocatives, such as *John, Mummy* (when used as calling signals);
(iii) Other, such as interjections (e.g. *oh, yugh*), and phrases that perform a variety of social functions, such as greeting and thanking (e.g. *hello, sorry, ta*);
(iv) Problems, i.e. cases where it is unclear to which category to assign a minor sentence, or where it is uncertain whether a one-word sentence is major or minor.

Other types of Minor sentence (full or partial Stereotypes) are handled under Section A (see 2.5.2).

2.7.2* Major sentences can be analysed in two main ways:

(i) in terms of the layers of structure they contain, and the types of grammatical rule which apply to them;
(ii) in terms of their communicative type.

No structural subdivisions are formally recognized at Stage I, but three main communicative sentence types are represented on the chart: *statements, questions* and *commands*. Because of the greater opportunity P has to use statements in clinical settings, more detail is given about types of sentence structure under that heading, especially at later Stages. The columns for handling questions and commands contain a less detailed breakdown into types. The only reason for this is convenience—P samples containing fewer instances of questions and commands, and thus requiring less room to be available on the chart. It is not being suggested that questions and commands are somehow less important than statements; they are simply less used.

2.7.3 Very little information about formal sentence structure is available at Stage I—clear syntactic patterns emerge only throughout Stage II (see below). Even the identification of word classes (parts of speech) is a tentative matter at Stage I, hence the use of inverted commas around the category labels—to remind the analyst of the ever-present danger of reading in normal adult values to P's immature sentences.

Under Statements, the chart contains 4 categories:

(i) 'N'—items that seem to be used as nouns, such as *boy, houses, car;*
(ii) 'V'—items that seem to be used as verbs, such as *walk, running, gone;*
(iii) Other, such as adjective-like items (e.g. *nice, big*), adverb-like items (e.g. *asleep, quickly*), pronoun-like items (e.g. *him*), etc.
(iv) Problems, where it is unclear to which category an item should be assigned—whether formal (N, V etc.) or functional (statement, question, command).

Only one category is represented under Questions and Commands at Stage I:

'Q' stands for question-words, such as *what, where, when, how;*
'V' stands for verbs used as imperatives, such as *jump!, stop!*

2.7.4 Two common difficulties should be anticipated:

(i) There may be ambiguity between 'V' as statement and 'V' as command, at this stage. Intonation does not always suffice to distinguish the uses, and context may not be clear. In such cases, the sentence is assigned to the Problems category (cf. above).
(ii) The use of intonation as the marker of a questioning attitude has no place on this chart, which recognizes only the formal categories of morphology and syntax. 'Intonational questions' are an interesting stage in prosodic development, however, and there is a place for them on the prosody profile (see 4.5.4).

2.7.5 As part of profiling procedure, any morphological structure in major sentence elements is noted in the word-column (see futher, 2.10). For example, *boys* is analysed as 'N' and *plural; walking* is 'V' and *ing*. Pronouns, when they occur as single-element sentences, are also marked at Stage III (see futher, 2.11.2), in view of their unique developmental significance.

Stage I may therefore be summarized as follows:

Stage I (0:9–1:6)	Minor		Responses			Vocatives	Other	Problems
	Major	Comm.	Quest.		Statement			
		'V'	'Q'	'V'		'N'	Other	Problems

A typical Stage I pattern would be as follows:

Stage I (0:9–1:6)	Minor		Responses 40			Vocatives 1	Other 4	Problems
	Major	Comm.	Quest.		Statement			
		'V'	'Q'	'V' 2		'N' 24	Other 11	Problems

This was a language-delayed 3½-year-old, who in this sample (talking about a picture) produced 82 sentences in reply to T''s stimuli. Over half were Minor sentences—40 Responses (entirely made up of *yes* and *no*), 1 Vocative and 4 Others (all interjections). The rest of the profile showed a marked nominal bias (24), with few verbs; the 11 Others were mainly Pronouns (*him, that*). There were no cases of Command or Question sentences—which may have been no more than a consequence of the sampling situation (though the likelihood of a genuine weakness here needs to be borne in mind). In view of the way in which verbs play a central role in the subsequent development of clause structure, an important remedial goal was to produce a more balanced profile at Stage I, by working on 'V', in both Statement and Command functions.

2.8* Stage II runs from about 1½ to 2 years of age. It is a stage at which sentences characteristically contain two elements—but the emphasis is not so much on sentence length as on the qualitative range of sequences which can be used. At this stage, there is enough formal variation in sentence patterning to justify the introduction of the main analytical levels in the grammatical theory we use: *clause, phrase* and *word*.

2.8.1* At the level of the clause, five constituent elements are recognized; these elements may be represented by complex constructions in the adult language, but at Stage II they tend to be single words or simple phrases.

(*i*) *Subject* (S)   A selection of clauses containing a Subject plus one other clause element is as follows:

daddy go/   *man* in bus/   *a man* eating/   *him* happy/
S   S   S   S

Somewhat more complex sentences, but still with a 2-element clause structure, are:

a window broke/   *he* started to laugh/   *what I said* hurt/
   S   S   S

(ii) Verb (V)   A selection of clauses containing a Verb plus one other clause element is as follows:

kick ball/   man *go*/   he *walking*/   him *jump*/   *see* man/
   V   V   V   V   V

Somewhat more complex 2-element clauses containing a Verb clause element are:

the man *came*/   he *has gone*/   I *sat down*/   he *wanted to go*/   *did* he *go*/
     V   V   V   V   V . . . V

(iii) Object (O)   A selection of clauses containing an Object plus one other clause element is as follows:

kick *ball*/   want *car*/   see *me*/   eating *a cake*/
   O   O   O   O

Somewhat more complex examples include:

ask *him*/   stop *that car*/   say *what you want*/   look at *my photo*/
   O   O   O   O

(iv) Complement (C)   This less well-known element is defined as the part of the clause governed by a form of the verb *to be* (or a few other verbs, such as *become, seem*), or following where, in immature speech, such a form would be expected. A selection of clauses containing a Complement plus one other clause element is as follows:

him *happy*/   that *a ball*/   is *nice*/
   C   C   C

Somewhat more complex 2-element clauses include:

don't be *clever*/   be *quiet*/   might be *a fire*/   seems *OK*/
     C   C   C   C

(v) Adverbial (A)   A selection of clauses containing an Adverbial plus one other element is as follows:

man *there*/   happy *now*/   going *in car*/   jump *soon*/
   A   A   A   A

Somewhat more complex 2-element clauses include:

go *in the garden*/   run *where you like*/   come *tomorrow morning*/
   A   A   A

2.8.2 The combination of clause elements recognized at Stage II of the LARSP chart are located in the columns under Statement, Question and Command, as follows:

		Clause	
VX	QX	SV	AX
		SO	VO
		SC	VC
		Neg X	Other

Thus, SV means: 'a clause containing the elements S and V (though not necessarily in this order)'. While we have printed the combinations in the order in which they normally occur, the possibility of alternative element orders need to be borne in mind (e.g. *tickle daddy,* where the child wants daddy to tickle HER—*daddy* is plainly intended as Subject, despite the abnormal element order). A negative particle (Neg) may also be used as a separate clause element at this stage, and this is noted separately.

Examples of each of these structures are:

SV	daddy going, me want, the man is walking
	S V S V S V
SO	man ball (where context makes it plain that the sense is 'man
	S O kick ball', or the like)
	that boy a cat (= 'that boy has a cat')
	S O
SC	man happy, him very clever
	S C S C
Neg X	not car, running no, no a man (a negative word, accompanied
	Neg X X Neg Neg X by any other clause element)
AX	man there, man in garden, there a car, going now
	X A X A A X X A
	(X = any other clause element)
VO	kick ball, see a man, want new car
	V O V O V O
VC	is nice, am tired, be a big aeroplane
	V C V C V C
Other	all-gone teddy, car broken
	?C/?V ?S S ?V/?C
QX	where man, what doing, gone where
	Q X Q X X Q (X = any other clause element)
VX	sit there, put in box (where context makes it clear that a
	V X V X command sense is involved)

An expected clause distribution in a small sample at Stage II was as follows:

Clause				
VX **2**	QX **4**	SV **12**	AX	**9**
		SO **1**	VO	**10**
		SC **6**	VC	
		Neg X **3**	Other	

SV and VO are both well represented, and there is a strong AX. SC, SO and Neg X represent immature structures whose use will die out if subsequent development is normal. Normally developing children would also have a few QX and VX in a conversational sample—even in such tasks as picture description (it is difficult to stop questions!). By contrast, the clause profile taken from a language-delayed child is given below, showing marked immaturity, an avoidance of verb constructions, an adverbial bias (largely due to over-use of *there*), and no sign of the initiative required to use QX or VX. Work on verb constructions (VO, then SV) would here be a priority.

Clause				
VX	QX	SV *1*	AX *18*	
		SO *7*	VO *1*	
		SC *8*	VC	
		Neg X *4*	Other *3*	

2.8.3* A clause element may take the form of a single word, as in *daddy go*.
$$\text{S} \quad \text{V}$$
But as language matures, the elements are more likely to be expanded as a string of words, or *phrase*. The process can be seen operating as follows:

	S	V
	man	go
	the man	is going
Phrases {	that very nice man	might be going
	that very nice man in a raincoat	doesn't want to keep on going
	etc.	etc.

If the string of words has a noun as its grammatical centre (*man* in the above), it is known as a *noun phrase;* if it has a verb as its centre (*go* in the above), it is known as a *verb phrase*. There are also *adverbial phrases*, illustrated by

V	A	
go	tomorrow	
	in the morning	} Phrases
	in the morning of the match	
	etc.	

At Stage II, sentences may consist solely of two-element phrases—in other words, lacking any clause structure. As is clear from the above examples, there are far more possibilities of phrase sequences than in the case of clause structure; hence only the most commonly occurring patterns are given separate mention in the Phrase box on the profile chart, as follows:

DN	VV
Adj N	V part
NN	Int X
PrN	Other

DN (Determiner + Noun)　*the boy, my house, that car, some eggs,*
　　　　　　　　　　　　　D　N　　D　N　　　D N　　D　　N

Adj N (Adjectival + Noun)   *nice box, big boy, three dogs*
                             Adj N   Adj N   Adj N
N N (Noun + Noun)   *mummy's key, mummy daddy, railway station*
                     N   N   N   N   N   N
Pr N (Preposition + Noun)   *in box, for John, under table*
                            Pr N Pr N   Pr   N
VV (Verb + Verb)   *want go, wanna go, make jump*
                    V   V   V   V   V   V
V part (Verb + particle)   *come in, sit down, shut up*
                           V part V part   V part
Int X (Intensifier + some other phrase element)   *very nice, really big, all*
dirty   Int X   Int X Int
  X
Other, e.g. Pr Pron (Preposition + Pronoun)   *to me, in that*
                                              Pr Pron Pr Pron
         Pr Adv (Preposition + Adverb) *in there, on here*
                                       Pr Adv Pr Adv

A typical Stage II phrase pattern, using a small sample from a normal 20-month-old, was as follows:

Phrase			
DN	*10*	VV	*3*
Adj N	*6*	V part	*7*
NN	*6*	Int *X*	*1*
PrN	*11*	Other	*5*

All categories are represented, though several were restricted lexically (for example, Det is *that, my*, with no sign of the articles). By contrast, the following phrasal profile was taken from a language-delayed 3-year-old, using the same type and size of sample:

Phrase			
DN	*4*	VV	
Adj N	*1*	V part	
NN		Int *X*	
PrN	*2*	Other	*21*

The high Other category is noteworthy, due to an over-reliance on 'empty' forms such as *in there* and *on that* (see further, 5.9.4); but there are also gaps, especially in the verb phrase. Remediation here would try to produce a more balanced profile, and also ensure that each category covered a good lexical range (a high figure opposite Adj N, for example, is only a sign of progress if a varied set of adjectives is used).

2.9* In mature speech, as we have seen (2.8.3), clause elements may be expanded by phrases; but at Stage II this has not taken place. The process of introducing phrases into the clause is not an easy one for the child, as the task is one of learning to handle grammatical *hierarchy*—the existence of different levels of structuring within one sentence. To increase the 'size' of the sentence *daddy go* to *my daddy go* does more than simply 'add a word'—it adds an extra layer of grammatical structure, as can be seen from the conventional way of representing these things:

my daddy   go

Clause   S   V
              ‾‾‾‾‾‾‾

Phrase   D   N

The ability of the child to introduce phrases into his clause structure is therefore plotted separately on the LARSP chart. As the process seems to take quite a while before it is firmly established, it is plotted in two places. The first stage of phrasal expansion seems to occur towards the end of Stage II, and is indicated on the chart by a 'transitional line' between Stages II and III. Along this line are plotted those phrasal expansions which take place in *two*-element clauses. A little further down, between Stages III and IV, a similar transitional line is used to plot those phrasal expansions which take place in *three*-element clauses. (There is no separate tally made of phrasal expansions in clauses of four or more elements.) The two transitional lines appear as follows:

X + S:NP	X + V:VP	X + C:NP	X + O:NP	X + A:AP

XY + S:NP	XY + V:VP	XY + C:NP	XY + O:NP	XY + A:AP

The formulae are to be interpreted in the following way:

$X + S: NP$ A 2-element clause has its Subject expanded by a Noun Phrase (or clause); the remaining element in the clause is not further identified, but is labelled X. Examples include:

a man walk   *the man there*

  S   V   (i.e. S + X)   S   A   (i.e. S + X)
 ‾‾‾‾‾‾   ‾‾‾‾‾‾

 D   N   (i.e. NP)   D   N   (i.e. NP)

           ∴ X + S: NP   ∴ X + S: NP

To profile these sentences each step in the analysis is transferred to the profile chart, viz.

Stage II clause structure—a mark opposite SV and AX;
Stage II phrase structure—a mark opposite DN, for each sentence;
Stage II transitional line—a mark opposite X + S: NP, for each sentence.

The result would appear as follows:

Clause				Phrase	
VX	QX	SV ✓	AX ✓	DN ✓✓	VV
		SO	VO	Adj N	V part
		SC	VC	NN	Int X
		Neg X	Other	PrN	Other
X + S:NP ✓✓	X + V:VP	X + C:NP	X + O:NP	X + A:AP	

The same principles apply to the other formulae, viz.

X + V: VP A 2-element clause has its Verb expanded by a Verb Phrase
(of any type), the remaining element being referred to as X, e.g.

man is running
X + V: VP

X + C: NP A 2-element clause has its Complement expanded by a Noun
Phrase (clause, or adjectival construction), the remaining element being
referred to as X, e.g.

is a man   *it nice to eat*
X + C: NP   X + C: NP

X + O: NP A 2-element clause has its Object expanded by a Noun Phrase
(or clause), the remaining element being referred to as X, e.g.

kick a ball
X + O: NP

X + A: AP A 2-element clause has its Adverbial expanded by an
Adverbial Phrase (or clause), the remaining element being referred to as X,
e.g.

go in there
X + A: AP

XY + S: NP A 3-element clause has its Subject expanded by a Noun
Phrase (or clause), the remaining elements being referred to as X and Y
respectively, e.g.

the man go town
  S: NP X   Y   (= XY + S: NP)

XY + V: VP A 3-element clause has its Verb expanded by a Verb Phrase,
the remaining elements being referred to as X and Y respectively, e.g.

he is going now
X V: VP Y   (= XY + V: VP)

XY + C: NP A 3-element clause has its Complement expanded by a
Noun Phrase (clause, or adjectival construction), the remaining elements
being referred to as X and Y respectively, e.g.

he is a doctor
X Y + C: NP

XY + O: NP   A 3-element clause has its Object expanded by a Noun Phrase (or clause), the remaining elements being referred to as X and Y respectively, e.g.

he is kicking the ball
X   Y   + O: NP

XY +A: AP   A 3-element clause has its Adverbial expanded by an Adverbial Phrase (or clause), the remaining elements being referred to as X and Y respectively, e.g.

the man went to town
X   Y + A: AP

A normal distribution of transitional line structures is shown in the following example: all elements are expanded, but there is a marked bias towards the expansion of postverbal elements.

| X + S:NP **7** | X + V:VP **15** | X + C:NP **4** | X + O:NP **12** | X + A:AP **11** |

| XY + S:NP **5** | XY + V:VP **21** | XY + C:NP **6** | XY + O:NP **18** | XY + A:AP **8** |

By contrast, the transitional lines of a language-delayed P are given below, showing verb-phrase gaps, and an abnormal Subject expansion bias (perhaps due to a concentration of remedial work on this area). Work on the expansion of postverbal elements would seem to be an urgent remedial goal.

| X + S:NP **8** | X + V:VP **1** | X + C:NP | X + O:NP **2** | X + A:AP **2** |

| XY + S:NP **11** | XY + V:VP | XY + C:NP **1** | XY + O:NP | XY + A:AP **1** |

In the extreme case of 'telegrammatic speech', there would be no expansions at all, and these lines would stay blank.

2.10* Word-endings with a grammatical function begin to be used from the beginning of Stage II, and a tentative order of emergence is given in the Word column at the right of the chart. The various abbreviations have the following application:

-ing   e.g. kick*ing*, runn*ing* (but not when given a nominal use, as in *Smoking is forbidden*);

pl   e.g. cat*s*, hors*es*, m*i*ce, mous*es* (i.e. *any* plural form, whether regular or irregular, correct or incorrect);

-ed   e.g. I walk*ed*/ r*a*n/ s*aw*/ went*ed* (i.e. any simple past tense form, whether regular or irregular, correct or incorrect);

-en   e.g. I have tak*en*/ g*one*/ took*en*/ walk*ed* (i.e. any past participle form, whether regular or irregular, correct or incorrect);

3s   e.g. walk*s*, goe*s*, *is*, *has* (i.e. any third person singular present tense form, whether regular or irregular, correct or incorrect);

gen   e.g. boy*'s*, men*'s*, cats*'*, boys*'s* (i.e. any genitive form of a noun, whether regular or irregular, correct or incorrect);

n't   e.g. ca*n't,* does*n't,* better*n't* (i.e. the contracted negative form, whether correct or incorrect);

'cop   e.g. he'*s* happy, I'*m* a salesman (i.e. the contracted form of the copula verb (see 2.11.2), whether correct or incorrect);

'aux   e.g. he'*s* coming, I'*m* walking, you'*s* kicking (i.e. the contracted form of the auxiliary verb (see 2.11.2), whether correct or incorrect);

-est   e.g. bigg*est,* nic*est,* best*est, best* (i.e. the superlative form of an adjective or adverb, whether regular or irregular, correct or incorrect);

-er   e.g. bigg*er,* nic*er, better,* mor*er* (i.e. the comparative form of an adjective or adverb, whether regular or irregular, correct or incorrect);

-ly   e.g. quick*ly,* slow*ly,* big*ly* (i.e. the ending used to mark an adverb word class, whether correct or incorrect).

(Incorrect forms are also marked in the 'error' box at Stage VI (see 2.14.2).)

On the left, below, there is an illustration of an expected Word profile pattern, taken from a normal 3-year-old; on the right, a comparable sample, taken from a language-delayed 5-year-old, displaying, in particular, a marked weakness in verb forms.

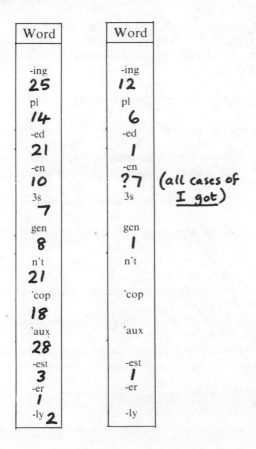

Word-endings play only a minor part in the expression of grammatical relationships in English, and remedial work in this area should not proceed without considering the other (phrasal and clausal) factors involved. In the above case, for example, the weakness in verb endings is part of a more general difficulty with the verb phrase, and appropriately broad teaching strategies (*not* just focusing on the endings) would need to be devised.

2.11* Stage III runs from about 2 to 2½ years of age. It is a stage at which sentences characteristically contain 3 elements; but it also subsumes certain developments at phrase level which are unrelated to the matter of clausal complexity.

2.11.1 The following combinations of clause elements are to be found in the Statement, Question and Command columns:

SVC   *that is interesting   the man is a doctor   I was sorry to go*
           S   V   C   S   V   C   S   V   C

SVO   *the man kicked the ball   I saw him   I know what he did*
           S   V   O   S   V   O   S   V   O

SVA   *the man went to town   the man is over there   I came before you*
           S   V   A   S   V   A   S   V   A

Neg XY   *no man come   not go bed   go car no*
          Neg X   Y   Neg X   Y   X   Y   Neg
(i.e. a Negative word with two other elements of clause structure, labelled X and Y respectively)

VCA   *is happy now   will be a chair in a minute*
          V   C   A   V   C   A

VOA   *kicked the ball into the goal   seeing him there*
          V   O   A   V   O   A

VO$_d$O$_i$ i.e. the distinction between a direct and an indirect Object, as in: *gives a letter to the man   passed it to me   gave me it*
                  V   O$_d$ O$_i$ V   O$_d$ O$_i$ V   O$_i$ O$_d$

Other,   e.g. VAA   *going there now   went to town in a bus*
                  V   A   A   V   A   A
                SO$_d$O$_i$ *that man a letter to that man* (i.e. 'gave' a letter)
                    S   O$_d$ O$_i$

QXY   *what you doing   where man gone*
          Q   X   Y   Q   X   Y
(i.e. a question-word with two other elements of clause structure, labelled X and Y respectively)

VS(X)   *is he, is he going, are they kicking a ball*
          V   S   V- S   -V   V- S   -V   X
(i.e. a question formed by inverting the order of Subject and the first part of the Verb Phrase; if there is a third element of clause structure, it is labelled X)

VXY   *put that there, give the man a letter*
          V   X   Y   V   X   Y

(where the context makes it plain that a command sense is intended; the various possibilities under X and Y are not subclassified on the chart)

let XY   *let me go*   *let the man fall*   *let's kick the ball*
         let X Y   *let* X   Y   *let*   X   Y

do XY   *do stop that*   *don't do that*   *don't talk to him*
         do X   Y   *do*   X Y   *do*   X   Y

(i.e. a form of the verb *do* when used as a command)

An expected Stage III clause profile, for a small sample, was as follows:

V X Y **1** *let X Y* *do X Y* **2**	Q X Y **4** VS(*X*) **1**	SVC **6** SVO **20** SVA **15** Neg *X Y* **3**	VCA **2** VOA **1** VO$_d$O$_i$ **1** Other **1**

By contrast, the following profile was taken from a language-delayed child of 4, who was beginning to use Stage III clauses, after a long period of training at Stage II. He is showing some strength in SVO, but his Subject position is still weak, as can be seen from the right hand side of the box, and there were some funny structures under Other (e.g. *in town is in the morning*—AVA). There was no sign of any Question or Command structures.

V X Y *let X Y* *do X Y*	Q X Y VS(*X*)	SVC SVO **7** SVA **2** Neg *X Y* **2**	VCA **3** VOA **6** VO$_d$O$_i$ Other **6**

2.11.2 At phrase level, several of the phrasal constructions in use at Stage II expand into three element phrases, the most common being:

D Adj N   *the big box*   *a nice car*
         D Adj N   D Adj N
Adj Adj N *nice big car*   *big red train*
         Adj Adj N   Adj Adj N
Pr D N   *in the box*   *behind the table*
         Pr D   N   Pr   D   N

There are many other, less common types, such as N Adj N (e.g. *mummy's big car*), Pr D Pron (e.g. *in this one*). These would be noted under Other, in the Stage III Phrase box.

Apart from this, this box contains three other forms whose importance to normal development is central.

Pron (Pronoun) refers to any item which can replace a Noun Phrase, such as *he, I, that, one, something*. A distinction is made between the personal pronouns (P) and other sorts of pronouns (O). The personal pronouns are

I, you, he, she, it, we, they, along with their grammatical variants (e.g. *he saw him*).

Cop (Copula) refers to the verb *be,* in any of its forms, when it is the only verb in a clause, as in *he is happy, he is a doctor.*

Aux (Auxiliary) refers to the small set of verbs which alter the tense, aspect or mood of the main verb. They are divided into two types: *modal* (M) auxiliaries are *can/could, will/would, shall/should, may/might, must, dare, need, ought, have to,* along with their negative forms; the other (O) auxiliaries are the various forms of *be, have, do* when used along with a main verb (e.g. *he is going   he has gone   he might come   he can go*).

$$\text{Aux}^o \qquad \text{Aux}^o \qquad \text{Aux}^m \qquad \text{Aux}^m$$

A typical Stage III phrase profile, in a small sample, would contain a scattering of 3-element phrases, a fairly large number of pronouns (of both kinds), and strongly-developing copula and auxiliary systems (including both modal and other verbs). One such profile is illustrated here:

D Adj N **5**	Cop	**6**
Adj Adj N **1**		**9**
Pr DN **8**	Aux_O^M	**11**
Pron_O^P **18 10**	Other	**3**

By contrast, a typical language delay profile will have few or no auxiliaries and copulas, and a strong pronominal bias (i.e. the pronouns being used as an 'escape route' to avoid having to use noun phrases), as in the following case:

D Adj N **2**	Cop	
Adj Adj N		
Pr DN **1**	Aux_O^M	
Pron_O^P **24 16**	Other	**11**

In view of the importance of the auxiliary and copula verb systems to the subsequent development of more complex clauses (and especially clause sequences), careful attention would need to be paid to this area of the chart in planning remedial work. Also, the tendency to use pronouns in place of noun phrases would need early correction, if longer sentences were not to become increasingly ambiguous (e.g. *boy saw man* and *he went . . .*).

2.12* Stage IV runs from about 2½ to 3 years of age. It is a stage at which clauses characteristically contain 4 or more elements. At phrase level there is a comparable growth in complexity, but here the stage is more notable for the development of new types of phrasal construction.

2.12.1ʳ The following combinations of clause elements are to be found in the Statement, Question and Command columns:

SVOA   *the man kicked the ball into the goal   he put it there*
          S   V   O   A   S V O A

SVCA   *he will be ready at three   the boy was sad when he fell*
          S   V   C   A   S   V   C   A

SVO_dO_i *he gave me a letter   I gave a book to the man*
          S   V O_i O_d S V O_d O_i

SVOC   *he made me happy   I thought him an idiot*
          S   V   O   C   S   V   O   C

AAXY   *he went to town yesterday   soon I arrived in Africa*
          X   Y   A   A   A X   Y   A

(i.e. a clause containing two adverbials, along with two other elements of clause structure, labelled X and Y respectively)

Other,   e.g. SVAAA *I went to town yesterday in a bus*
                    S   V   A   A   A
                SVOCA *I found him interesting at first*
                    S   V   O   C   A

QVS   *where is he   what is he doing*
          Q   V   S   Q V- S -V

(i.e. a question-word along with subject-verb inversion)

QXY+   *what daddy doing   where man is going   why gone now*
          Q   X   Y   Q   X   Y   Q   X   Y

(i.e. a question-word accompanied by 2 other clause elements, and *lacking* the inversion required in mature speech); if there are more than 2 other elements, the + sign becomes relevant, e.g.
    what you putting in garden now
    Q   X   Y   Z   W
                 +

would simply be noted under QXY+, without further specification.

VS(X+)   *have they kicked the ball into the garden*
          V-   S   -V   X

(i.e. a subject-verb inversion followed by more than one other element of clause structure)

tag   *he's coming/ isn't he   he is/ is he*
                  tag   tag

(i.e. a VS construction 'tagged' onto the main clause; its own internal structure is logged elsewhere on the chart, under VS, Pron, etc.)

+S   *you sit down   all you children come here*
          S   V   S   V   A

(i.e. a command with the Subject expressed; all such patterns are logged under this heading, regardless of the number of clause elements they contain)

VXY+   *give me that now, put the cow in the box quickly*
            V   O   O   A   V   O   A   A
         = V   X   Y   +   V   X   Y   +

(i.e. a command verb with more than 2 other elements of clause structure accompanying).

A typical Stage IV clausal profile, in a normally-developing child, is given below. The Other box is mainly taken up with variations using Adverbials.

+ S 1	QVS 4	SVOA 25	AA XY 7
	Q $X Y$ +	SVCA 9	Other 18
V $X Y$ +	VS(X+) 13	SVO$_d$O$_i$ 4	
	tag 12	SVOC 3	

By contrast, there are several imbalances and gaps in the following Stage IV profile taken from an ESN(M) child of eight: the immature Question pattern should be noted; the Other figure this time is also due to the persistence of immature construction (e.g. *he is the soldier happy now*—?SVCCA). Consolidation of the SVOA basic pattern would be an early remedial goal.

+ S	QVS	SVOA 2	AA XY 1
	Q $X Y$ + 4	SVCA	Other 8
V $X Y$ +	VS(X+)	SVO$_d$O$_i$	
	tag 1	SVOC	

2.12.2 There is considerable variety in the range of structures at phrase level in Stage IV.

NP Pr NP   *the man in a hat   a little car with a red roof*
            NP   Pr   NP   NP   Pr   NP
(i.e. a sequence of 2 noun phrases linked by a preposition, the second postmodifying the first; each NP is then separately profiled as DN, D Adj N, or whatever)

Pr D Adj N   *in the big box   behind the red car*
            Pr D Adj N   Pr   D Adj N

cX   any phrasal construction introduced by a coordinating conjunction (c), usually *and,* as in:
            and me   and the boy;
            c   X   c   X
if the construction labelled X has any internal structure, this is profiled elsewhere on the chart in the usual way, e.g. *the boy* in the last example would be profiled as DN)

XcX   two phrasal constructions linked by a coordinating conjunction, usually *and,* as in:
            boy and girl, a big man and a red car;
            X   c   X   X   c   X
as previously, if the X construction has any internal structure, it is profiled elsewhere on the chart in the usual way (e.g. *a big man* would be D Adj N)

Neg V   *he isn't going   he is not running*
            Neg   V   Neg   V
(i.e. a negative word *within* the verb phrase—as opposed to its earlier status as a particle external to clause structure, in Stages II and III)

Neg X   *he has a pencil/ not a pen*
                    Neg   X
(i.e. a negative word within a phrase other than the verb phrase)
2 Aux   *he may be going, I have been kicked*
                  2 Aux   2 Aux
(i.e. any sequence of two auxiliary verbs within the verb phrase)
Other,   e.g. Pr D Adj Adj N *in that big red box*
                  D Adj Adj N *a big fat pig*

A typical Stage IV phrasal profile, in a normally-developing child, is given below. The Other box is quite large, due to a wide range of constructions being attempted, and the XcX construction is usually quite prominent.

NP Pr NP	16	Neg V	12
Pr D Adj N	8	Neg *X*	1
c*X*	4	2 Aux	4
Xc*X*	15	Other	24

Language-delayed children who have reached Stage IV usually display weaknesses in the verb phrase and in phrasal coordination (apart from a few fixed phrases, such as *mummy and daddy*); problems of short-term memory also usually keep the noun phrases fairly short—hence few NP Pr NP.

NP Pr NP	2	Neg V	1
Pr D Adj N		Neg *X*	
c*X*	3	2 Aux	
Xc*X*	2	Other	3

2.13* Stage V runs from about 3 to about 3½ years of age. The primary characteristic of this stage is the development of complex sentence formation, through the stringing together of clauses, and the embedding of one clause within another. The most notable development in the structure of the chart, therefore, is the addition of a column wherein the type of connecting word can be noted (headed *Conn.*).

2.13.1 Four types of connecting word are recognized. Because *and* is the most frequently used connector, it is tallied separately. Other coordinating conjunctions (c)—*or, but,* etc.—are grouped together. Subordinating conjunctions (s), such as *when, although, because, which,* are also grouped together. And other words or phrases whose use is primarily connective are placed under the heading of Other—for example, *well* and *so*. A typical spread of figures for a child producing fluent connected speech at this Stage is as follows (though these figures cannot be properly interpreted without reference to the connectivity patterns under the heading of Clause—see below):

2.13.2 Two main classes of clausal connection are recognized on the chart: coordination (Coord.) and subordination (Subord.). The most detailed set of distinctions is given for Statements:

Coord 1   two clauses linked by *and* or c; each clause is then profiled separately, in the usual way, e.g.

> *the man saw a dog and the lady saw a cat*
>   Clause   *and*   Coord Clause
>   ∴ *Coord 1 marked at Stage V*

(The two SVOs are then profiled at Stage III, and the remainder of their structure handled at the appropriate places on the chart.)

Coord 1+   more than two clauses linked by *and* or c; each clause is then profiled separately, in the usual way, e.g.

> *I came and he went and we all laughed*
> Clause *and* Clause *and*   Clause
>   Coord 1   Coord 2   ∴ *Coord 1 + marked at Stage V*

Subord A 1   a clause containing an adverbial element which is itself a clause, and marked as subordinate by the use of s; each clause is then profiled separately, in the usual way, e.g.

> *he arrived when it was dark*
> S   V   _____A_____
>   ∴ *Subord   A 1   marked at Stage V*
>   s   S   V   C
>   etc.

Subord A 1+   a clause containing at least two adverbial clauses; each clause is then profiled separately, in the usual way, e.g.

> *he arrived when it was dark and when it was raining*
> S   V   _____A_____ *and* _____A_____
>   Subord Clause 1   Subord Clause 2
>   ∴ *Subord A 1 + marked at Stage V*

Subord S   a clause containing a Subject (S) element which is itself a clause; once this point has been noted, and the subordinating conjunction marked in the Connectivity column, the two clauses are profiled separately, in the usual way, e.g.

what I said was important
   S   V   C
—————

∴ *Subord S*   *marked at Stage V*
  s S V

         etc.

Subord C a clause containing a Complement (C) element which is itself a clause; profiling procedure is as above, e.g.

that is what I wanted
S V   C
    —————

     ∴ *Subord C*   *marked at Stage V*
      s S   V

   etc.

Subord O a clause containing an Object (O) element which is itself a clause; profiling procedure is as above, e.g.

he knew what I wanted
S   V   O
     —————

     ∴ *Subord O*   *marked at Stage V*
    s S   V

  etc.

Comparative a clause containing a grammatical marker of comparison, such as *bigger than, as big as.* The internal clause structure of the comparative element is not profiled in detail. For example,

he is bigger than I am
S V   C
     —————

  ∴ *Comparative*   *marked at Stage V*
  (no further analysis)

Questions and Commands also permit the use of coordination and the various types of subordination and comparison. On the LARSP chart, instances of clausal coordination are grouped under one heading, and other forms are grouped under *Other,* as follows:

Question Coord   *when is he coming and why is he*
Question Other   *what did you do after you fell off*
Command Coord *sit down and shut up*
Command Other *sit down when you're ready*

A typical illustration of a normal Stage V pattern is as follows: the bias towards coordination is notable, and certain types of subordinate clause are plainly more frequent than others:

and **29** c **10** s **19** Other	Coord. Other **1**	Coord. **1** Other **2**	Coord. **1 30** 1+ **8** Subord. A **1 14** 1+ **3** S **1** C **1** O **14** Comparative **2**

By contrast, the following pattern is taken from a language-delayed child of 7, who was beginning to make inroads into Stage V, but who was struggling with all but the simpler constructions. The lack of correspondence between the figure for *and* and that for Coord is notable: P had developed the habit of introducing many sentences with *and,* whether or not a coordination meaning was intended. An important remedial aim was therefore to eliminate this habit, to bring *and* more under control and to establish his comprehension of the strategies underlying coordination and subordination.

and **15** c s **3** Other	Coord. Other	Coord. Other	Coord. **1 4** 1+ Subord. A **1** 1+ S C O **3** Comparative

2.13.3 A small range of clauses may also be introduced as part of noun-phrase structure, as one of the means of postmodifying the head noun. A clause may occur once (1) or several times (1+):

Postmod. clause *the man who saw me is outside*

$$\underline{S \qquad\qquad} V \quad A$$

Clause 1   ∴ Postmod. clause 1 at Stage V

s   V   O

etc.

there's the car which you drove and which was bumped
S V   C

Clause 1   Clause 2   ∴ Postmod. clause 1 + at Stage V

The remainder of the grammatical analysis is transferred to the profile chart in the usual way: the main clause is first profiled, then the clause structure of the postmodifying clause(s), and then the phrase and word structure belonging to each clause.

Postmod. phrase 1+   *the man in the garden in a hat*
NP   Pr   NP   Pr   NP

Postmod.   Postmod.   ∴ Post mod. phrase 1
phrase 1   phrase 2   at Stage V

(A single case of a postmodifying phrase can be profiled at Stage IV, under NP Pr NP (see 2.12.2); the present section of the chart deals only with sequences of *more than one* (postmodifying) prepositional phrase.)

2.14* Stage VI runs from about 3½ to about 4½ years. Two quite distinct processes seem to be operating, and these are handled under the symbols + and −. + stands for *new* types of construction, not previously used at earlier stages. − stands for *errors* made as the child completes the learning of constructions found earlier on the chart.

2.14.1 Because of the limited amount of research which has been done into this age range of grammatical acquisition, only a small selection of new constructions is cited. On the left of the + box are listed two constructions from within the noun phrase:

Initiator
all the cows, both the men
  I D N   I   D N
(i.e. the item(s) preceding the determiner in a noun phrase; a mark is placed on the chart next to Initiator, and the 3-element phrase (in this pair of examples) is added to the total at Stage III (under *Other* in the phrase column).
Coord
John/ the butcher   look at that car/ the red Ford
 NP   NP   NP   NP
NP Coord at Stage VI refers to cases where two noun phrases are coordinated without any formal marker of the coordination present.

In the centre of the + box, just one heading is used, referring to more complex kinds of verb phrase than those listed earlier in the chart. For example, the verb phrase *he might not go* contains both an Auxiliary and a Negative: each of these would have been assigned to their respective categories at Stages III and IV; but the fact that they have been used together in the same verb phrase would not have been noted. Their cooccurrence is therefore logged separately under Complex VP at Stage VI.

On the right of the + box, three further kinds of Clausal construction are noted:

Passive
the cat was bitten by the dog   he was kicked
  S   V   A   S   V
These constructions will be profiled as SVA and SV accordingly, but to leave them as that would be to miss a major observation concerning their grammatical function—that they are passive in form, as opposed to active. All such sentences are therefore marked under Passive, in addition to the remainder of their analysis.
Complement.
he is loath to do it   I'm good at maths
 S V   C   S V   C

(Such structures illustrate a more complex form of complementation than that handled earlier in the chart; the existence of this more advanced form is therefore noted under *Complementation* (abbreviated to *Complement.*) at Stage VI, with no more detailed analysis taking place at this stage.

how/what

how nice it is, what a pretty dress (she was wearing)
    C   S V   C   S   V

These are clauses with exclamatory function, identified as such by the use of the 'question-words' *how* or *what* with normal SV element order following (unlike questions, where a question-word would be followed by SV inversion, as in *what is he doing*). The mark at Stage VI identifies this special function, with the remainder of the grammatical analysis being profiled earlier in the chart in the usual way (SVC, Pron, Cop, etc.).

The category of *Other* is available at Stage VI for any further constructions which develop during this period.

2.14.2* In the right-hand part of Stage VI (the 'error box'), a classification is made of the main kinds of mistakes which a child makes in his grammatical learning at this point. The terms 'error' and 'mistake' are of course from the point of view of the adult language target; from the child's 'viewpoint', they may be logical extensions of principles previously learned (as when the plural *-s* is generalized to irregular forms, such as *mouses, sheeps*). Errors, in the LARSP approach, are therefore viewed positively—as indications of progress, whereby the child is attempting to sort out an area of grammar which poses particular difficulty.

The main divisions in the error box reflect those used further up the chart, using the main distinctions between Connectivity, Clause, Phrase and Word. Each instance of an error is marked once, in the appropriate place.

(a) Under Connectivity (Conn.) are placed the main types of problem encountered during the learning of connecting words:

and	*he broke his arm and the ladder slipped* (where *and* is being used in place of a more appropriate subordinating marker);
c	*he broke his arm but the ladder slipped;*
s	*the ladder slipped cos he broke his arm* (which suggests that the comprehension of the conjunction is only partial).

Other problems of clausal connectivity (for example, inadequate or ambiguous cross-reference between clauses using pronouns) are noted as they arise, under *Other*.

(b) Clause errors are classified under three headings:

element omitted (∅): *he put on table* (i.e. O omitted), *he came in and the ball* (V omitted);
element order (⇆): *the dog the man chased* (i.e. SOV, where SVO is expected), *the cat bit the dog* (where P meant the reverse);
concord: *he are coming, they kick himself* (i.e. failure of the Subject to agree in number with another element);

(c) Phrase errors are classified in terms of whether they are located in the

noun phrase (NP) or the verb phrase (VP). Within the NP, they are further classified in terms of whether they affect determiners (D), prepositions (Pr) or personal pronouns (Pron^p). Within the VP, they are further classified in terms of whether they affect modal or other auxiliaries (Aux^m and Aux^o respectively), or the copula.

D (= the wrong form of determiner is used), e.g. *much tree, an information;*
D Ø (= a determiner has been omitted), e.g. *I see man;*
D ⇆ (= a determiner is in the wrong place), e.g. *man a there;*
Pr (= the wrong preposition is used), e.g. *he kicked the ball on the goal;*
Pr Ø (= a preposition has been omitted), e.g. *he kicked the ball the goal;*
Pr ⇆ (= a preposition is in the wrong place), e.g. *he kicked the ball the goal into;*
Pron^p (= all errors in the use of personal pronouns), e.g. *him going, he is going* (in a context where 'she' is required);
Aux^m (= all errors in the use of modal auxiliaries, whether of substitution or of order), e.g. *he must* (= 'can') *jump, he jump can;*
Aux^o (= all errors in the use of other auxiliaries, whether of substitution or order), e.g. *he be going, he do going, he going is;*
Aux Ø (= all omissions of an auxiliary, whether modal or other), e.g. *he going;*
Cop (= all copula errors, not further subclassified), e.g. *he sad, he be sad.*

Any phrase errors which do not fall within the above categories are logged under *Other.*

(*d*) Word errors are those affecting morphological structure in respect of the use of the inflectional endings used earlier in the chart. Two main categories are recognized: errors in the *noun* (N), and errors in the *verb* (V). These are further subdivided, in terms of whether *regular* (reg) or *irregular* (irreg) items are involved.

N$_{irreg}$ (= the wrong form of an irregular noun), e.g. *mouses, sheeps;*
V$_{irreg}$ (= the wrong form of an irregular verb), e.g. *tooken, wented;*
N$_{reg}$ (= the wrong form of a regular noun), e.g. *boyses;*
V$_{reg}$ (= the wrong form of a regular verb), e.g. *singinging, I walken;*

Other types of morphological problem are logged under *Other.*

(*e*) It is often not possible to be sure to which category an error belongs. Errors which cannot be clearly related to one or other of the above are therefore logged separately, under *Ambiguous,* e.g. *he did fought* (= 'he fought?' 'did he fight?' 'he did fight?').

2.14.3 A typical example of the patterns of development shown in the Stage VI error box is given below, taken from a normal 4-year-old. The errors are not particularly frequent, but they are fairly widespread. The point to be noted is that, in normal development, these errors would be sorted out quite quickly, so that another sample taken 6 months later would show a dramatic reduction in number and range of errors.

(−)

Conn.	Clause	Phrase				Word	
	Element	NP			VP	N	V
and	∅ **2**	D **3** Pr **2** Pron^P		**8**	Aux^M **2** Aux^O **4** Cop **1**	*irreg* **6**	**4**
c	←→	D∅**3** Pr∅					
						reg	**1**
^{s} **2**	Concord **4**	D ←→ Pr ←→			∅		

Compar. adj. 2	Ambiguous **5**

By contrast, the following error box is taken from a comparable sample produced by a partially-hearing child of 9, whose overall grammatical level was around Stage III. The frequency with which certain categories cause problems is quite abnormal, and there are several Other errors. An analysis of all these errors would generally bring to light the range of constructions which P was finding particularly difficult, or where there had been overgeneralization from a pattern introduced into a teaching situation.

(−)

Conn.	Clause	Phrase				Word	
	Element	NP			VP	N	V
and	∅ **8**	D **2** Pr **11** Pron^P **21**			Aux^M Aux^O **18** Cop **11**	*irreg* **7**	**12**
c	←→ **7**	D∅ **15** Pr∅ **10**					
						reg **1**	**2**
^{s}	Concord **10**	D ←→ **7** Pr ←→ **2**			∅ **26**		

Adj. position 3 **X̶c̶X̶ 3**		
Adv. position 2 **Neg V 3**	Ambiguous **21**	

2.14.4 Finally, a point of profiling procedure in relation to the error box should be noted. Errors are tabulated only when there is an indication of correct learning taking place elsewhere in the sample. For example, a determiner error would be counted as such only if there was evidence of the correct use of determiners somewhere else in the sample. Without this constraint, there would be no way of limiting the notion of 'error', and it would cease to be useful as an index of progress. For instance, if 'error' means simply 'everything that is wrong from the adult point of view', then in the following Stage I sentence, a whole host of 'errors' would have to be recognized: P points to a picture of a car and says *càr!*. But it would be absurd to penalize the child for 'failing' to say an SVC construction, a Copula, a Determiner, a Pronoun, and so on (assuming a full form of this sentence to be *That's a car*). A child can hardly be penalized for *not* doing something which is only to be expected at a later stage of linguistic development. The error box is therefore restricted to those problems where there are reasonable grounds for thinking that P should be able to cope with the construction, and the evidence is in P's 'trial and error'—the simultaneous occurrence in a sample of a correct use of a category (*at least one* correct instance) and its incorrect use. Only in these circumstances are the incorrect uses listed at Stage VI.

For example, P says *want car*. Would this be profiled as D 0? If there is no sign of any correct D use elsewhere in the sample, the answer is no. Conversely, if P has used a determiner correctly, at least once, then the omission would be logged at Stage VI.

2.15* Stage VII has little real assessment value, in that it has been so little studied in acquisition research. There may indeed be other stages within it, as the child's learning proceeds from age 4½ until it is wholly adult in character. It is not even clear at what age grammatical learning comes to be commensurate with the adult system (though the onset of puberty is often cited). As a consequence, LARSP lists only some of the more advanced structures at Stage VII, and provides only a mnemonic concerning the importance of three general acquisitional themes—*discourse, syntactic comprehension* and *style*.

(a) Discourse refers to the development of advanced strategies by which a child alters the structure of his sentences to take into account the needs of the listener, and to build up more complex themes in his connected speech (or writing).

A (= adverbial) connectivity (= more advanced ways of joining sentences than those introduced at Stage V), e.g. *as a matter of fact, however, unfortunately, actually;*
comment clause (= a parenthetic clause introduced into connected speech), e.g. *you see, you know, I mean;*
emphatic order (= an alteration in the normal word order of a clause, for reasons of emphasis), e.g. *Jòhn my 'name is/;*
it (= a construction in which a clause is split into two parts, the first part being introduced by an 'empty' *it*), e.g. *it was in the garden that I saw him* (from 'I saw him in the garden');
there (= a construction introduced by an 'empty' *there*), e.g. *there were lots of people in the garden* (from 'Lots of people were in the garden').

The category of *Other* is available for any further constructions noted in a sample which have no place elsewhere on the chart.

(b) Syntactic comprehension is a mnemonic label, intended to prompt T to scan the data for any cases where syntactic production seems to be in advance of comprehension. For example, P might be attributing a particular meaning to an NP-VP-NP pattern, which is not that of the adult language—he might assume that the first NP always 'does' the action, for instance (which would mean he would fail to comprehend, and perhaps misuse passive constructions, as in *the dog was bitten by the man*). Any such developments would be noted in an ad hoc way in this section.

(c) Style is also a mnemonic label, intended to prompt T to scan the data for any cases where P seems to be developing alternative grammatical varieties, or styles. A distinction between formal and informal speech is common, and—depending on circumstance—one might expect to find the influence of

television, advertising, religion and other such contexts. Any special forms associated with these varieties would be noted in an ad hoc way in this section.

2.16* LARSP provides only a brief indication of the patterns of grammatical interaction between T and P, but this is enough to show the importance of this dimension in assessment and remediation. The patterns are displayed in Sections B, C and D of the chart, which correspond to the main steps in a clinical linguistic interaction. If we take a piece of dialogue such as the following, these steps can be clearly seen:

T	'what's thàt 'called/	*Stimulus*
P	a càr/	*Response*
T	'good bòỳ/	*Reaction*

The patterns of T stimulus and P response are classified in Section B. The nature of any further reaction provided by T is classified in Section D. In Section C is classified any Spontaneous sentences on P's part—those used without any grammatical stimulus from T. Problematic and Unanalysed sentences, in the sense of Section A (cf. 2.5) are not logged under Sections B or C.

2.16.1 T's stimuli are noted on the left-hand side of Section B. They are classified into two broad types: *Question* and *Other* (this distinction being drawn on grammatical grounds).

Question stimulus e.g. 'what's he dòing/, 'is he in the cár/, he's rùnning/ ísn't he/.
Other stimulus e.g. 'that's a càr/, 'put that dòwn/, mhṁ/, he's rúnning/ (NB the rising intonation is not counted as a *grammatical* question).

2.16.2 P's responses are classified in terms of whether they are *normal, abnormal* or *problematic* (i.e. unclear which category to use). In addition, any response which is a repetition of the whole or part of T's stimulus is noted in the box headed *Repetitions*.

(a) There are only two types of abnormal grammatical response:

Zero response (symbolized as Ø) where T gives P time to respond to a stimulus, but P says nothing.
Structural abnormality where the grammatical pattern of P's response does not match that required by T's stimulus, as in *T 'what's he dóing/ P yès/*. It should be noted that a decision concerning structural abnormality is made independently of semantic considerations. For example, P replied *wheels* to the stimulus *where's the man driving;* this was a semantically relevant thing to say, but it did not fit the syntactic requirements of this stimulus, which are to have some kind of adverbial as response.

(b) There are several possible ways of responding normally:

Minor e.g. *yès/, thànks/, mhṁ/* (i.e. the use of a minor sentence to an appropriate grammatical stimulus).

Full major e.g. *I can 'see a càr/, 'that is a bòy/* (i.e. the use of a complete major sentence appropriate to the grammatical stimulus).

Elliptical major e.g. *T 'where is he góing/ P to tòwn/* (i.e. the use of an incomplete, but grammatically predictable major sentence). Elliptical responses are then classified in terms of the number of *clause* elements they contain, viz.

(i) a single clause element (logged under Elliptical major 1), as in the example above, where *to town* is a single Adverbial element;

(ii) two clause elements (logged under Elliptical major 2), as in *T 'where is he gòing/ P 'going to tòwn/*

V   A   Elliptical major 2

(iii) three or more clause elements (logged under Elliptical major 3 +), as in *T 'who 'bumped the càr/ P 'John 'did yèsterday/*

S   V   A

Elliptical major 3

Reduced major e.g. *T 'what's hàppening/ P 'man in gàrden/* or *'man sàd/* (i.e. the use of a sentence where elements have been left out due to the immaturity of P's speech; because they are not formally derivable from T's stimulus, they are not elliptical, in the sense of the above).

(c) Repetitions would include such cases as *T: 'what's hàppening/ P: hàppening/*. The response would have its grammatical type classified under normal or abnormal as above, and *in addition* a mark would be placed in the repetitions box. It should be noted that, to count as a repetition, the prosodic pattern of the response ought to be the same as that of the stimulus.

2.16.3 P's first sentence in reply to a T stimulus counts as his *response*. Any additional sentences he may use (along with any used *without* a preceding T stimulus) are called *spontaneous*, and are classified in Section C. The same categories are used here as in Section B (apart from the Abnormal categories, which cannot by definition apply). Thus, the monologue below would be analysed in the following way:

T	'what can you sée/	
P	I 'see màn/	*Full major response*
	'him 'going tòwn/	*Full major spontaneous*
	'going on bùs/	*Elliptical major 2, spontaneous*
	'going on 'bus with làdy/	*Elliptical major 3, spontaneous*
	'that nìce/	*Reduced major, spontaneous*
	gôsh/	*Minor, spontaneous*

2.16.4 T may react to P's response in several ways, and a detailed account would need to make reference to semantic, social and other factors. From the grammatical point of view, the range of reactions can be reduced to five main types (allowing, as always, for a category of *Problems*):

General (= reactions that are structurally unrelated to P's sentence), such as *yes, good boy, m;*

Structural (= structurally related reactions), as when P's sentence is given a grammatical expansion, e.g. *P it càr/ T it's a càr/;*
Zero (= the absence of any reaction from T, who proceeds to a new stimulus directly);
Others (= reactions unrelated to the interaction), as when T talks to self while preparing a new stimulus or task;
Repetitions (= a repeat of the grammatical form that P used), as when T attempts to get a more accurate production—as in many pronunciation drills.

2.16.5 The conversational interaction in a half-hour sample between a normal 4-year-old and her parent is analysed in terms of Sections B, C and D below.

A	Unanalysed				Problematic		
	1 Unintelligible **2**	2 Symbolic Noise	3 Deviant		1 Incomplete	2 Ambiguous	3 Stereotypes

B	Responses				Normal Response						Abnormal		
						Major							
	Stimulus Type	Totals	Repetitions	Elliptical 1	2	3+	Reduced	Full	Minor	Structural	∅	Problems
	21 Questions	**21**		**10**	**5**			**2**	**4**			
	46 Others	**44**		**6**	**2**	**1**		**24**	**11**		**2**	

| C | Spontaneous | **181** | **2** | **8** | **3** | | | **2** | **168** | | | | |

D	Reactions		General	Structural	∅	Other	Problems
		65	**36**	**1**	**28**		

This profile has several important features. There is a predominance of Other Stimuli (i.e. relatively few direct questions). The child's language is strongly spontaneous, with minor, full major and elliptical major sentences in use (elliptical replies being an important feature of conversational style). Some zero responses are used (even normal children don't reply, sometimes!). Along the Other line, the total Stimuli and the total Responses do not coincide, because there were 2 Unintelligible sentences used, which were transferred to Section A directly (cf. 2.5). The majority of the child's spontaneous speech are full major sentences. There are a couple of self-repetitions (not uncommon in play situations). An important point is the nature of maternal reactions: this particular mother does not intervene all that often (about once in every 4 of the child's sentences), but when she does her reactions are either zero (i.e. she does not react at all to what has just been said, but proceeds to a new stimulus directly) or general (in this case, predominantly *mhm*).

There is a marked contrast between this profile and the following one, taken from a half-hour therapy session with a language-delayed child of the same age.

A	Unanalysed				Problematic		
	1 Unintelligible **8**	2 Symbolic Noise	3 Deviant		1 Incomplete	2 Ambiguous	3 Stereotypes

B	Responses							Normal Response					Abnormal		
							Major								
	Stimulus Type		Totals	Repetitions	Elliptical			Reduced	Full	Minor	Structural	∅	Problems
					1	2	3+						
82	Questions	**44**	**3**	**4**			**10**	**1**	**21**	**8**	**30**	
12	Others	**2**							**2**		**10**	

C	Spontaneous	**4**						**4**						

D	Reactions		General	Structural	∅		Other	Problems
		46	**14**	**30**			**2**	

Here, T finds himself having to use predominantly Question stimuli, to elicit any response from P (the 12 Other stimuli produced 10 zero responses). Even so, there is a marked reluctance to reply, and many of the replies are monosyllabic (21 minors, mainly *yes* and *no*) or structurally abnormal or reduced. There is hardly any spontaneous speech. T reacts explicitly to almost every one of P's sentences, either with a general reinforcing phrase (such as *that's right*) or (more commonly, in view of the structured nature of the interaction) with a structurally related reaction.

2.17* Along the bottom line of the chart, certain summarizing features of the sample can be added.

(a) The total number of P sentences can be obtained from the Totals given in Sections B and C (or, alternatively, from the transcript, if these sections have not been analysed). A half-hour sample generally produces between 100 and 200 sentences.

(b) Each instance of Stimulus + Response (+ Reaction) is called a conversational *turn*. The mean number of sentences P uses within each turn is calculated by dividing his total sentences by the Total T stimuli. For example, in the interaction profiles above, the normal child produces 246 sentences in relation to 67 stimuli: her mean number of sentences per turn is therefore 246/67 = 3.7. The language-delayed child produces 90 sentences in relation to 94 stimuli—a mean of 0.96.

(c) Mean sentence length can only be obtained from the transcript, by counting the number of words (defined conventionally as items in the transcript with space on either side), and dividing this by the total number of sentences. For example, in one sample the following numbers obtained:

Words in sentence	No. of instances	Total words
1	54	54
2	34	68
3	9	27
4	4	16
5	0	0
6	1	6
	102	171

Mean sentence length is therefore 171/102 = 1.68—very low indeed.

2.18 As pointed out at the beginning of this chapter, there has been no concern in the above exposition to recommend a particular way of working through the types of information presented on the LARSP chart. How one proceeds is to a large extent determined by the kind of P one is working with. But in all cases, it is crucial to devise a way of laying out a grammatical analysis so that the information obtained from the various grammatical scans is clearly indicated. A common procedure is to represent a sentence analysis vertically, with the types of grammatical information labelled on the left (as a reminder to check that everything has been taken into account). For example:

a man is walking

Conn.				
Clause		S	V	
Phrase		D N	Aux	v
Word			3s	ing
Expansions	X + S: NP	X + V: VP		

2.19 While for the purposes of illustration the various examples of clinical analysis in this chapter have all been of children, it should be borne in mind that the LARSP approach is equally available for analysing the grammatical difficulties of adults. Similarly, while the examples in the chapter have for the most part been devoted to the analysis of speech production, the procedure can also be used for the analysis of samples of writing or signing, and for the study of other modes of language use (comprehension, imitation).

2.20 Lastly, it is recognized that the method of exposition used in this chapter has been artificial in one major respect. By outlining one Stage at a time, only a partial picture could be given of the difficulties manifested in the various samples. It will therefore be helpful to provide a complete analysis of a clinical sample, so that the integration of the various steps can be observed. An extract from one such sample is given below: it is taken from an initial assessment session with a 4½-year-old, who had been referred for treatment of a language delay with accompanying problems of nonfluency. A LARSP analysis was made of a 15-minute conversation with T, while playing with a toy house and farm.

T	have you 'got one like thát/	*referring to carpet*
P	nò/	
T	nòt like 'that/	
	'what 'colour's yóurs/	
P	me – 'me ain't gòt cárpets/	
T	you 'haven't got cărpets/	
	'what dò you have/	
P	'just	
T	thìs/	*referring to a bathroom mat*
	thìs sort of thíng/	

P	yēah/
T	well this ìs a sort of cárpet/ ìsn't it/
P	nò/
	lòok/
T	oh it's beaùtifully 'soft/ ìsn't it/
P	thàt/ can 'go upstàirs/
T	yès/
	thàt's trúe/
P	(*1 syll*) dòwnstairs thére/
T	wêll/
P	'what's thàt/
T	'what do you thìnk it 'is/
P	oh is –
	is 'that a mìrror/ ìsn't it/
T	it ìsn't a mírror/ be'cause you 'can't sèe your'self/ –
	it's a 'sort of cùpboard/ .
	I 'think 'that one 'goes a'gainst the wàll/ –
	can you 'put it a'gainst the wáll 'somewhere/ —
P	(5 *sylls*)
T	'will it ŏpen/
P	nò/
T	yès it wíll/
	'that's grèat/
P	Ì can – Ì can pút/ – tòys in thére/
T	if we hàd any tóys/ –
	but we 'don't 'seem to hàve any 'toys in thís 'house/ —
	'what 'toys hàve yòu 'got/
	'what's your bèst 'toy/
P	ràcing 'car/
T	a ràcing 'car/
P	yèah/
T	and 'does it have a tràck to gó on/
P	nó/
T	'what do you dò with your 'racing 'car/
P	(just) 'pull it on the flòor/
T	oh I sèe/
	you 'put it on the flòor/
	and 'how does it 'go alòng/ —
	do you 'have to wínd it/ – or whàt/
P	[wɒ . wɒnt] àh/
	the dìnner/ *referring to a cooker*
T	what còlour is your 'racing 'car/ —
	'tell me abòut your 'racing 'car/
P	whíte/
T	it's whĭte/
	and 'does it have a mán in it/
P	yèah/
T	and 'how fàst does it 'go/
P	rèally 'fast/ —

	(we'll have) some méat/	*referring to toy piece of meat*
T	'that's a vêry 'large 'piece of 'meat/ ìsn't it/ –	
	I should 'put that in the 'cupboard till we 'have vìsitors/	
P	yéah/ – –	
	and thàt one/	*referring to pan*
T	it'll 'go in 'that cùpboard/ – –	
	'that'll be a nìce 'cupboard to 'put it in/ –	
	we 'haven't 'got a frìdge/ hàve we/ –	
	dó you 'have a 'fridge/	
P	yèah/ – –	
	is . whìte/	
T	it's a whìte ʲfridge/	
P	yèah/	
	réally whìte/	

The LARSP profile related to this extract is given on p. 49. It illustrates a clear picture of grammatical delay, though there are complications arising out of phonological and lexical factors (see further below). A commentary on the profile produces the following points:

Section A   Only 9 unintelligible sentences are found in the whole sample, but several of them are quite lengthy 'attempts' at complex structures (analysed further below).

Sections B/C/D   P's spontaneous total is low, compared with that for responses (mean number of sentences per turn is only 1.1). Minor sentences constitute over half his responses to Question stimuli. Elliptical responses are quite high, and full major responses to Questions are low—suggesting a considerable dependence on T's question structure. Structural abnormality and zero responses are also in evidence, suggesting difficulties in P's comprehension and attention.

Stage I   One-element sentences constitute half the total number of sentences in the sample—an extremely high proportion. There are no cases of 'V', perhaps indicative of an expressive verb weakness in spontaneous speech.

Stage II   This is fairly thin, presumably because Stage III structures are (apparently) well-established. There are no S expansions in the transitional line between Stages II and III.

Stage III   There is an apparently strong basic clause structure; but in fact it is rather stereotyped, due to P's overuse of a small set of verbs. Of 100 verb tokens in the sample, *be, got* and *go* constitute 60 per cent, with only *do* and *put* being comparable (a further 13 per cent). These are fairly 'empty' verbs, from a semantic point of view (see further, Chapter 5).

Phrase structure, at this stage, seems to be developing normally; but in fact, the high Aux figure is suspect, due to the frequency with which P uses *can* (one-third of all Aux cases) and a tendency to use Aux elliptically (e.g. *I ain't, it do,* and in tags) and not in full verb-phrase structure. The copula is also generally contracted (in two-thirds of cases). In the Word column, absence of *-ed* and a thin use of *-ing* (along with some errors at Stage VI) also suggests that there is an underlying verb weakness.

Subject expansions between Stages III and IV are few, and those used do

| Name | Shane P. | | Age | 4;6 | | Sample date 25.11.80 | Type | Free play, toys (15 mins.) |

A | **Unanalysed** | | | | **Problematic**

A	Unanalysed				Problematic			
	1 Unintelligible **9**	2 Symbolic Noise	3 Deviant		1 Incomplete **4**	2 Ambiguous	3 Stereotypes **7**	

B Responses

				Normal Response						Abnormal		
					Major							
			Repet-	Elliptical			Red-	Full	Minor	Struc-	∅	Prob-
Stimulus Type		Totals	itions	1	2	3+	uced			tural		lems
66 Questions		**59**		**15**	**4**	**2**		**2**	**32**	**4**	**5**	
44 Others		**36**	**1**	**8**				**12**	**14**	**2**		

C Spontaneous **39** | | **7** | **6** | | | **5** | **11** | **10** | | |

D Reactions **95**

	General	Structural	∅	Other	Problems
	30	21	43	1	

Stage I (0;9–1;6)

Minor | Responses **42** | Vocatives | Other | Problems

Major | Comm. | Quest. | Statement | | | | |
| | 'V' **2** | 'Q' **3** | 'V' | 'N' **10** | Other **5** | Problems |

Stage II (1;6–2;0)

Conn.	Clause				Phrase		Word
	VX	QX	SV **6**	AX **4**	DN **20**	VV **1**	
			SO **1**	VO	Adj N **1**	V part **2**	-ing **5**
			SC	VC **1**	NN	Int X **1**	pl **5**
			Neg X	Other	PrN	Other **4**	-ed

Stage III (2;0–2;6)

X + S:NP	X + V:VP **3**		X + C:NP	X + O:NP **2**	X + A:AP **2**	
VXY	QXY **2**	SVC **14**	VCA **1**	D Adj N **5**	Cop **15**	-en **7**
let XY		SVO **12**	VOA **1**	Adj Adj N **1**	Aux$_O^M$ **8** **7**	3s **31**
do XY **5**	VS(X)	SVA **16**	VO$_d$O$_i$	Pr DN **6** **20**		gen
		Neg XY	Other	Pron$_O^P$ **16**	Other **4**	

Stage IV (2;6–3;0)

XY + S:NP **7**	XY + V:VP **13**		XY + C:NP **5**	XY + O:NP **7**	XY + A:AP **7**	
+ S	QVS	SVOA **1**	AAXY	NP Pr NP	Neg V **8**	n't **7**
	QXY +	SVCA	Other	Pr D Adj N	Neg X	'cop **10**
VXY +	VS(X+)	SVO$_d$O$_i$		cX **1**	2 Aux	'aux **1**
	tag **5**	SVOC	all tags	XcX **1**	Other	-est

Stage V (3;0–3;6)

and **3**	Coord.	Coord.	Coord. **(5)** **1**	1+	Postmod. **1** clause	1+	-er
c	Other	Other	Subord. A **1**	1+		clause **1**	
s **3**			S C O		Postmod. **1+** phrase		-ly
Other		Comparative					

| (+) | | (−) | |

Stage VI (3;6–4;6)

NP	VP	Clause	Conn.	Clause		Phrase			Word	
				Element		NP		VP	N	V
Initiator	Complex	Passive	and	∅	D	Pr **2**	Pron^P	Aux^M Aux^O Cop	irreg **1**	
Coord.	**7**	Complement.	c	⇄ **1**	D∅	Pr∅ **1**		**4** **1**		
		how what	s	Concord **3**	D ⇄	Pr ⇄		∅	reg	
Other			Adj. **1**					Ambiguous		

Stage VII (4;6+)

Discourse		Syntactic Comprehension	
A Connectivity	it		
Comment Clause	there **1**	Style	
Emphatic Order	Other		

| Total No. Sentences | **134** | Mean No. Sentences Per Turn | **1·1** | Mean Sentence Length | **2·6** |

not suggest that P can handle this area. In 75 cases where subjects were expected, he omitted it 30 times, used a pronoun 30 times, and used a noun phrase only 7 times. Of these, 4 were inverted order clauses (e.g. *where's the bathroom*), and 2 were semantically 'empty' (*that thing isn't open, that one's got a walking stick*). In short, there was only one clear case of subject expansion in the whole sample (*and the bath goes there*)—clearly indicating a problem. P may well be using tag questions as a means of avoiding subject expansion (cf. *'put that upstàirs/ còuldn't we/, 'bit tròuble hére/ wòn't I/*).

Stage IV   Apart from Neg V (largely in tags), the cut-off at Stage IV is quite clear. The cX is empty (*and that one*), the XcX may be a stereotype for him, and the attempt at a relative clause (Postmod. clause 1) went wrong (see further below). Tag questions are in use, but not very systematically, and his use of *don't they* might be stereotyped (it often fails to agree in number with the subject, e.g. *'that 'goes in thère/ dòn't they/*).

Stage V   There is a problem on P's horizon with this stage. He is beginning to use conjunctions (*and* and *cos* in particular). But, in the absence of clause development at Stage IV, and given the uncertain status of his verb phrase at Stage III, and his problems with subject expression (cf. above), this sign of 'progress' must in fact be viewed with concern. It is not possible to develop good clause sequence at Stage V without a solid clause and phrase structure from earlier stages. If allowed to continue unchecked, one might predict in due course the emergence of such sentences as *he kicked the man and can fall down*, with increasing ambiguity if the *and* sequence were allowed to continue.

There are already signs of P's difficulties as he attempts clause sequences. It is perhaps not a coincidence that the two main cases of unintelligible speech in the sample both involve *and*, viz.

> *some are doing (that) and – some (Verb)ing it in (there);*
> *(1 syll) gòt – one of thése/ 'got to 'put up a tràctor/ (2 sylls) 'put it in thère/ dòn't they/ – and and – (in) òut/.*

It should be noted also that as a sentence gets longer, it becomes increasingly reliant on context-dependent (deictic) items, such as *it, there, these, they, that*. This suggests that, as P tries to use his limited processing abilities for more advanced syntax, he 'gives up' on the lexical side, replacing specific items by 'empty' ones (cf. the adult P analysed in 5.10). He has a fairly marked tendency to do this in simpler sentences too (especially when referring to absent events, where the use of deictic forms is an inappropriate and unclear strategy).

P's attempt at a relative clause is *I don't want that what that is*—a normal developmental usage. It suggests, again, that he is 'willing' to take on Stage V constructions—but is not as yet competent to do so.

Follow-up session   This analysis was then used as input for a follow-up assessment session, in which various hypotheses about P's disability were tested. It was felt important to check on the extent of P's ability to handle the apparently weak areas of grammatical structure, viz. clause sequencing, verbs, and narrative abilities for absent topics. A puzzle which had emerged from the first session was P's fluency, which was within normal expectations (though previous case notes stated that he was very nonfluent). It was felt that if pressure were put on P to use the structures which were causing him problems, it might be possible to elicit this nonfluency. The aim of the follow-up session, therefore, was to push P as far as possible down the LARSP chart, to see whether the suspected weaknesses became more manifest as task complexity increased.

To this end, P was given the following four tasks:

(a) a comprehension task, of the 'do X and then do Y' type, proceeding to 'put X in Y and then put P in Q'. Conjunctions were progressively made more difficult *(before, when)*, and the number of clauses in the sequence was increased to three. P was also invited to give instructions to T along similar lines.

He did very well. He could handle sequences of two clauses with *and,* and two clauses with *when;* but he generally failed on *before.* When asked to instruct T, he used only *and,* but at one point spontaneously used a sequence of three clauses. However, his productions were strongly deictic (e.g. *put that on there)* and he became nonfluent several times (e.g. *and get open that . thingy/ . there/,* indicating drawled segments).

(b) LDA action cards were used to elicit verbs, and subject expansions, aiming for a move from 'he's Verbing' to 'a N is Verbing'. P had no difficulty naming the verbs, but he did have trouble with subject expansion. Asked to focus on the subject (using *who* questions, and by querying subject elements), he produced several non-fluencies, e.g.

> T   'is it a gírl 'sleeping/
> P   gìrl's/ fàther/ – whàt/ . ⓘ ìs/. what's 'gone in to (3 *sylls*)

Several *and*-sequences spontaneously emerged, from which it was possible to see signs of subject weakness on non-initial clauses—the omission of determiners, for example (e.g. . . . *and man's doing.* . .). On the other hand, several good noun phrases emerged (e.g. *and this boy is throwing his car/*). There is evidently a need to consolidate this element of structure. P made no attempt to use anything more complex than DN. It was felt unlikely that he could handle, say, D Adj N as Subject.

(c) LDA sequencing cards were used to elicit stories from P; then unstructured picture stimuli, to see whether this situation was more difficult for him.

There were several problems. P laid out the cards in an odd way, to begin with—vertically. They were in the right order, usually, but he insisted on talking about the final card first! On the whole he produced single-clause sentences; but he did attempt a few sequences, and in these cases several grammatical difficulties emerged, along with a fair amount of nonfluency (phrasal as well as segmental), e.g. (nonfluent utterance in italics):

> T   'what do you 'do in yòur 'garden/
> P   *'plant some* sèeds in thére/ *erm (plant) erm erm* 'put some wáter with it/ and – (1 syll) 'something ùp/ plànt 'comes 'up/

Examples of omitted clause elements in these sequences include:

. . . the *'flowers 'coming ùp/ cos the sùn/* (Verb Ø)
. . . *'fell ìn/ – 'push in the wàter/* (Subject *and* Object Ø)

Longer sequences become very confused, e.g.

'first there (look) – fishing 'rod/ – thèn 'look/ . 'catch the fish/ and 'then 'pushed it ìn/

—the point here being that in the penultimate clause, the omitted subject refers to the boy in the picture, whereas in the final clause it refers to the fish (who pulls the boy in). This kind of monologue must promote a great deal of unintelligibility.

This section also produced a couple of quite advanced structures, not previously noticed, viz. *which one did that called* (= 'what was it called') and *a knife was stuck in him* (an appropriately-used passive).

The unstructured picture stimuli were helpful, in that they elicited several unsuccessful attempts at Stage V structure, and underlined P's limitations. He was very reluctant to say more than one clause at a time; but when he did, it was regularly accompanied by nonfluency, false starts, and diminished prosodic strength. He repeatedly used a stereotyped *I don't know*. He mainly attempted *and*-sequences, but there was one interesting example of an attempt at a Subject-clause:

that thàt – b 'boot with . 'bird in/ . 'that is hìs 'shoe/.

He was in fact quite good at NP Pr NP, which is a foundation of later relative clause development (e.g. *the man in the garden → the man who is in the garden*). There could be a fruitful remedial path here, in due course.

(d) P was asked to tell stories about a favourite television programme, and to report on his morning's activities. This task demonstrated his problems very clearly, as the following sequences show. T has asked why the Incredible Hulk has been angered:

P	cos he gòt to/ – 'make . 'make him àngry/	*(NB Subject ∅)*
T	whàt made him 'angry/	
	whò made him 'angry/	
P	gìrl/	*(NB Det ∅)*
T	a gĭrl/	
	whỳ/	
	'what did she dò/	
P	thùmped her/	*(NB Subject ∅, and*
T	she did whát/	*changes Subject)*
P	thùmped her/	

The most marked piece of nonfluency in the whole session was when he was excitedly telling a story of what had once happened on a walk (there is erratic pitch, loudness and tempo control throughout):

m – m . m̀/ . my dàd 'went in the 'woods/ . a and mè/ – dád/ – mé/ – 'went in the wòods/ and 'we did 'saw a lòt of 'fox/ but my 'daā . but my 'dad . buT my 'dad kìlled it/

Conclusion   The picture of specific grammatical delay suggested by the LARSP profile is confirmed in the follow-up session. Several specific areas of difficulty are apparent, and seem to relate to P's nonfluency. One would in normal circumstances anticipate that the nonfluency would diminish as control over these structures improves; but P's particular difficulty with Stage V structures means that his learning here will take much longer than in normal development, and his nonfluency will probably persist for a longer period (and thus doubtless cause increasing concern). Immediate remedial grammatical goals would seem to be the following:

(i) the systematic building up of subject expansion, beginning with X + S: NP, and then XY + S: NP;
(ii) developing his use of structures (from the earlier stages) in contexts which he finds difficult, viz. absent or imaginary topics;
(iii) establish SVOA, but *without* reliance on deixis;
(iv) slowly build up Stage V, keeping clause structure very short to begin with, e.g. SV + SV; order-of-mention should be preserved (cf. 5.9.10), and reinforced by a clear sequence of reported events, e.g. 'X happened and then Y happened', where the activities are determinate and clearly causal.

2.21* While this is only a single illustration, it can be taken as typical of the way in which one proceeds from transcription to profiling to interpretation, and finally to remedial intervention. It should be noted, too, how necessary it is to refer back to the chart and to the transcription as one proceeds with the remedial discussion. The LARSP chart must not be seen in a vacuum: it is a summary of one's first systematic observations, and a guide to further observations. It is always necessary to interpret a chart in the context of the transcription on which it was based, and with reference to the other linguistic factors (phonological, lexical etc.) which identify P's disability.

3 PROPH

3.1* The segmental phonological profile known as PROPH ('*Pro*file of *Ph*onology') is essentially a presentation of the English sound system on a 2-page chart. To facilitate the compilation of the profile, a transcriptional page is added. To facilitate the interpretation of the profile, a separate 3-page section provides various suggestions about ways of summarizing the main patterns in the data.

3.2* The data base of the procedure is a sample of P's connected speech of up to 100 word-types (see further below). But there is no magic in the figure of 100. As with all profiles, one transcribes as much as is necessary to demonstrate a pattern in P's disability. Routinely, one might transcribe only a few dozen items to begin with, and profile these; the chart might then be sufficiently full to indicate the nature of the phonological problem. But if no clear pattern was emerging at this stage, a further sample would need to be taken. 100-word samples are usually enough to establish a pattern; but if necessary, the sample could be larger, using supplementary transcriptional pages. Sometimes, one has to be satisfied with what one can get!

Similarly, there is no obligation to use connected conversational speech, though this is what we aim for in the first instance. *Any* sample can be profiled (e.g. confrontation naming, the results of an articulation test, or the imitation of T speech). Information about sample type is indicated at the top of the page. Samples of different types should *not* be profiled together, unless some kind of typographical distinction is made on the chart.

3.2.1* Each word-type in the sample is assigned a line, and subsequent word-tokens of the same type are placed on the same line. For example, if P's first sentence were *daddy go* ['dædɪ 'gou], the transcription would appear as follows:

1 *daddy*   'dædɪ
2 *go*   'gou

If, later in the sample, P used these words again, they would be placed along the same lines as their first occurrence. If the later tokens were phonetically identical (to the analyst's ear) with the first, they would not be separately transcribed, but marked thus:

1 daddy   'dædɪ   ‖‖ ‖

(This would mean that, in the sample, P used this form 8 times—the original instance, plus a subsequent 7 instances.) Alternative pronunciations are listed separately along the same line (as far as space permits), e.g.

Phonological Profile (PROPH)

Name _____   Duration _____

Age _____   Sample date _____   Type _____

Accent conventions _____

Gloss	Transcriptions		Gloss	Transcriptions

Gloss	Transcriptions	Gloss	Transcriptions	Gloss	Transcriptions
1		41		81	
2		42		82	
3		43		83	
4		44		84	
5		45		85	
6		46		86	
7		47		87	
8		48		88	
9		49		89	
10		50		90	
11		51		91	
12		52		92	
13		53		93	
14		54		94	
15		55		95	
16		56		96	
17		57		97	
18		58		98	
19		59		99	
20		60		100	
21		61			
22		62		Problems	
23		63			
24		64			
25		65			
26		66			
27		67			
28		68			
29		69			
30		70			
31		71			
32		72			
33		73			
34		74			
35		75			
36		76			
37		77			
38		78			
39		79			
40		80			

Total word types _____   TTR _____

Total word tokens _____   Total problems _____

Repeated forms _____   Total unintelligible _____

Variant forms _____   Analysed:unanalysed _____

1   *daddy*   'dædɪ   'dægɪ   'dæ:ɪ

along with any indications of frequency, e.g.

1   *daddy*   'dædɪ   ‖‖   'dægɪ |

(This would mean that, in the sample, P used the form ['dædɪ] 4 times, and the form ['dægɪ] twice.)

The significance of this way of proceeding is to make it clear in the transcription just how much variability there is in P's production. Analysing the type and amount of variability in P's repeated use of words can provide important clues as to the nature of a disability and whether particular aspects of the sound system are undergoing a process of change.

It should be noted that the transcription treats grammatical variations as separate words, for the purposes of phonological analysis. For example, *cat* and *cats* would each have their own lines, as would *go, goes, going*.

3.2.2 In mature connected speech, some word-types turn up much more frequently than others, and this is often true of samples of phonological disability, especially where there is accompanying grammatical or semantic disorder. Generally, the distinction is drawn between the high frequency grammatical items (such as *the, that, and, yes, in, on, him*), and the lower frequency lexical items (such as *green, house, car, man*). While all P's words have to be considered in the overall evaluation of phonological disability (cf. the stress on comprehensiveness in 1.9), it is plain that difficulties with lexical items are going to cause P greater communicative problems than difficulties with grammatical items. A phonological profile needs to be able to reflect this distinction, upon occasion. Likewise, one needs to be able to handle the effects of having a single item (whether grammatical or lexical) turn up with abnormal frequency. For example, if P has 30 instances of a glottal stop replacing a target of final /-p/, it would be important to know whether these abnormal substitutions have occurred throughout several words, or whether they are there due to P's repeatedly using a single word with this abnormal substitution.

For these reasons, a separate section is provided on the transcriptional page for those items (grammatical or lexical) which T feels are going to turn up with abnormal frequency in the data, and which, if analysed in the routine way, would badly skew the profile. These items are placed in the unnumbered section, at the top of the page, along with any variations in pronunciation encountered in the data (as already described in 3.2.1.), e.g.

the ðə ‖‖ ‖‖ | də ‖‖   *it* ɪʔ ‖‖ ‖‖ ‖‖ ‖‖
a ə ‖‖ ‖‖ ‖‖ ‖‖ æ ‖‖   *and* æn ‖‖ ‖‖ n ‖‖ | nd |
him ɪm ‖‖ ‖‖ 'hɪm ‖‖ ‖‖   *there* dɛə ‖‖ ‖‖ ‖‖ dɛ: ‖‖

It should be emphasized that there is no theoretical motivation for the decision as to whether an item is placed in this section, or in one of the numbered lines below. T makes the decision based on his impression of the item's apparent frequency in the sample. Placing an item in the unnumbered section does not preclude its being profiled later; but we do leave the analysis of the items placed here until last, and often find that it is not particularly helpful to take them into account.

3.2.3 In cases where speech is unintelligible, the numbered section should not be used, as it is not possible to assign a target gloss to the word. On the other hand, it is important not to lose the information about the phonetic character of such unintelligible speech: its quantity may be an important aspect of assessment or indication of progress, and its qualitative range may provide fruitful guidelines for remediation. All unanalysable speech is therefore transcribed in the sample, and placed in the unnumbered section at the bottom of the chart, along with any tentative suggestions as to the meaning of the utterance, e.g.

```
        ?   'flaʊk lei
? horse  'nɔ:h
        ?   'spoun
```

Also in this section, one places utterances where an analysis in terms of word-level units is problematic, e.g. *gonna, dunno, I'll.* (Lexical compounds, such as *tea-bag, blackbird,* and so on, are taken as single lexical items, and assigned a numbered line.)

A complete sample of a language-delayed 4-year-old is given in 3.23 below.

3.3 Certain general principles governing the type of transcription used should be noted.

(a)* The initial descriptive statement is made using a phonemic model (for the profile's use of other models of analysis, see 3.21). However, because the phonological status of the phones in articulatory disorders is often unclear, it would seem premature to assign everything a phonemic status at the outset. On the other hand, it would be counterproductive (for a routine clinical tool) to aim for a maximally narrow phonetic transcription. Apart from the time-consuming nature of the enterprise, the quality of most clinical recordings would not permit it. PROPH therefore compromises, using a *broad phonetic* transcription—permitting a fairly specific representation to be given of the articulatory character of the phones used, and implying putative phonological status to these phones, but allowing for the possibility that such judgements may not on occasion be capable of being made. Thus, for example, if P pronounces the initial segment of *leaf* with a lateral fricative, this would be transcribed as [ɬ], and not phonemicized automatically to /l/; similarly, an open variant of the vowel in *men* would be transcribed as [ɛ̞]; and so on.

(b)* Because of recording fluctuations, limitations in the transcriber's ability, and a general indeterminacy in many P articulations (see further, 3.22.4), it is often not possible to do other than guess at the character of a phone. We therefore recommend use of the transcriptional conventions proposed by the working party investigating the phonetic representation of disordered speech, as reported in the British Journal of Disorders of Communication (December 1980). Chief amongst these, in our view, is the circle convention, to represent an element of uncertainty in the identification of a phone or phone type, as in ⓣ, Ⓒ or Ⓕ—standing for 'uncertain [t]', 'unspecified consonant' and 'unspecified fricative', respectively. We would attempt to profile items containing such circled symbols, allowing the circle to indicate on the profile chart the existence of our transcriptional indecision.

*(c)** The basis of the transcription is the phonological description of English used by Gimson, modified where necessary by standard IPA diacritics and symbols, and by the list of new symbols proposed by the working party referred to above. All items are judged as stressed or unstressed, in their connected speech context, and stress marks assigned to the items where needed (placed above and before the syllable). Only one degree of stress is recognized.

(d) Gimson's transcription is primarily concerned to characterize the type of English accent known as 'received pronunciation' (RP), and because of the intensive way in which this accent-group has been studied, we use it as the basis of PROPH's organization. But PROPH would hardly be useful if it were restricted to the articulation problems of RP speakers only! To bridge the gap between the RP model and the range of regional accents, therefore, page 1 of the procedure has a section headed *Accent conventions*. Under this heading is placed a note of those guidelines about P's accent (or that of his parents, peers, relatives) which will need to be taken into account in interpreting the profile chart. For example, P may drop all [h] phones from words which would have them initially in R.P. (*house, hurry* etc.). On the profile chart, therefore, he will have these words logged as lacking initial [h]. Now, if P comes from an accent area where [h] is expected initially, this [h]-dropping can be taken at face value, and remediation introduced at the appropriate time. But if he comes from an accent area where initial [h] is lacking, it would be unfair to penalize him for dropping the [h]. The purpose of *Accent conventions* is therefore to sensitize the profile user as to whether a sound is to be taken into account or not. In the present example, if it read

h- → ∅ (initial [h] is zero)

the analyst will note to pay no attention to the total of omitted [h]s on the chart. And similarly, for the following examples, all of which turn up quite commonly in regional speech:

-ing → ɪn   (*ing* endings are pronounced as [ɪn] not [ɪŋ])
əʊ → aʊ   (RP [əʊ] in e.g. *go* is produced as [aʊ]—as in Cockney, for
              instance)
-t- → -ʔ-   (RP medial [t] is replaced by a glottal stop, as in Cockney
              butter).

3.4 At the foot of page 1, certain general quantitative indices of the sample are recorded, namely:

(a) Total word types—i.e. the number of *different* words in the sample.

(b) Total word tokens—the number of words in the sample, i.e. including repeated instances of the same word.

(c) Type-token ratio (TTR)—the ratio of Types to Tokens, conventionally computed by dividing the total under *(a)* by the total under *(b)*.

(d) Repeated forms—the total number of phonetically identical word-tokens whose segments have been transferred onto the profile chart; for example, if P says *man* as [mæn] eight times, with no obvious phonetic variation, throughout the sample, this would be profiled as 8 cases of [m], 8 of [æ], and so on. The 7 'repetitions' would then be noted in the repeated forms

box. The total number of repeated forms should therefore always be referred to, in profile interpretation, to see whether any 'inflationary' element has entered the chart, due to P using certain words with exceptional frequency.

(e) Variant forms—the total number of word types on the transcriptional page, where the target word is represented by phonetically distinct alternatives; no separate count is made of the number of alternatives. For instance, in the following sample, there are three variant forms: *man, cat* and *boy:*

man	mæn men ‖ ma:		*dog*	dæg ‖‖	
cat	kæ: kæt		*boy*	bɒ bɔɪ ‖‖‖	

Noting the extent to which variant forms turn up in a sample could be an important indication of whether P's phonological system is undergoing change, and accordingly whether there is a good prognosis for remediation.

(f) Total problems refers to the number of items (types) which, for whatever reason, it has proved impossible to analyse in the sample.

(g) Total unintelligible refers to the number of word-like utterances (tokens) which it has proved impossible to interpret in the data (as opposed to those other problems where the target word is known, but a phonological analysis is wholly unclear).

(h) The ratio of *analysed* to *unanalysed* items (tokens) in the sample is likely to have some significance, as a measure of the extent to which the profile chart is a reasonable account of the sample as a whole. Obviously, if 60 words were in the sample, and only 30 were able to be analysed (the remainder being problematic or unintelligible), the picture is gloomier than if all 60 were analysable—and this will be reflected in the different ratios (30:60 as opposed to 60:60), the figure of 1 being the theoretical maximum.

3.4.1 Doubtless there are other statistical summaries that might be made of the transcriptional data, and other interesting ratios to be found. The above are only meant to be illustrative of the need to bear in mind some general characteristics of the sample, so that the profile description can be properly evaluated. It is too soon to say whether these ratios will have true clinical significance: too few cases have been analysed in these terms. With more precise longitudinal studies of phonological disability, however, we expect interesting findings to emerge.

3.5 The main part of the procedure is the 2-page classification of the segments which constitute the basis of the English sound system. These segments are classified in terms of (a) their distribution within syllables, and (b) their phonetic type.

3.5.1* The layout of the chart relates primarily to the distribution of segments within syllables. Syllables are analysed in the conventional way, as comprising a vowel nucleus, usually accompanied by a preceding consonant or consonant cluster, and often followed by a consonant or consonant cluster.

(a) Initial consonants (C-) are classified in the two left-hand columns in the upper part of the chart.

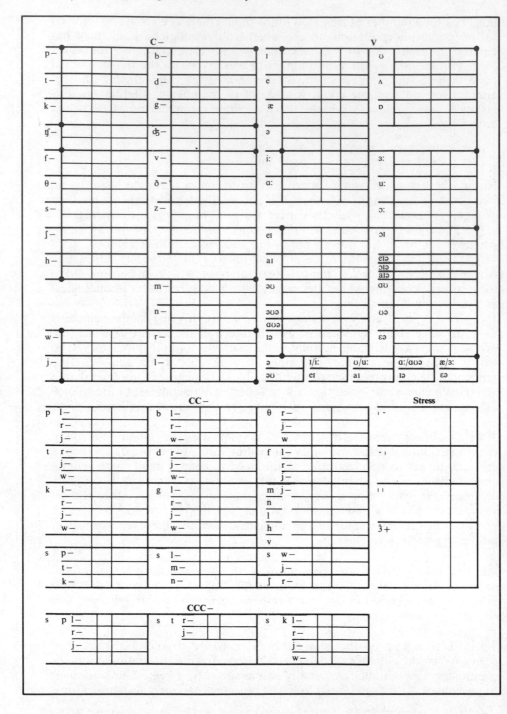

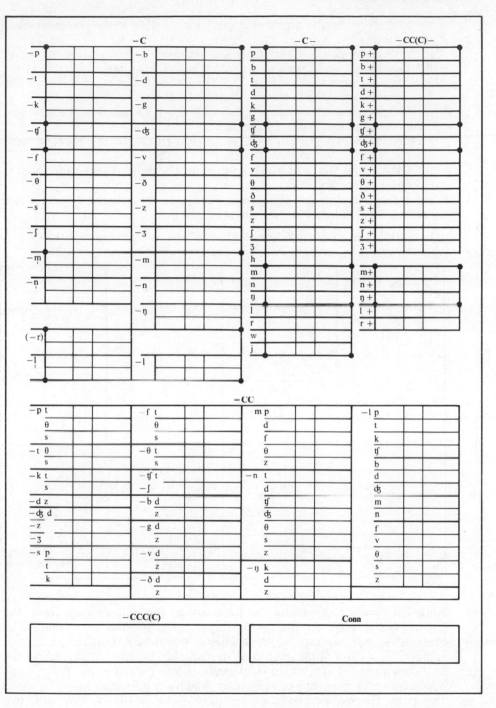

(b) Vowels (including diphthongs etc.) are classified in the two columns to the right of C-.

(c) Final consonants (-C) are classified in the two columns to the right of V.

(d) Consonants and consonant clusters whose distributional status in the syllable is uncertain (see further, 3.5.2) are classified in the two columns on the extreme right of the chart (-C-, -CC(C)-)

(e) Initial consonant clusters (CC-, CCC-) are classified in the left-hand columns in the lower part of the chart.

(f) Final consonant clusters (-CC, -CCC(C)) are classified in the right-hand columns in the lower part of the chart.

(g) The stress patterns of words containing 2 or more syllables are listed in the lower centre column.

(h) Information about phonological features of connected speech (see further, 3.12) is listed in the remaining section.

In outline, the chart therefore has the following organization:

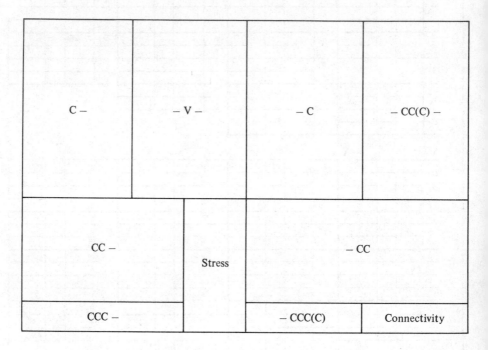

3.5.2 The profile procedure is to transfer the information from the transcriptional page to the profile chart, one syllable at a time. The consonants and vowels in monosyllabic words are transferred to the appropriate section of the chart directly: initial consonants, if any, under C-; final consonants, if any, under -C; vowels under -V-; and so on. Polysyllabic words, however, present a complication, which any profiling procedure has to anticipate. For our purposes, we see polysyllabic words as comprising two types:

(a) Those where the syllable division is quite clear, because there is a clear morphological boundary, as in *un/kind, walk/ing* etc. In such cases, each syllable is profiled in turn—*walk* [wɔ:k] would be C-, -V-, -C; *ing* would be -V-, -C; and so on. (Stress differences are also taken into account: see 3.8.)

(b)* polysyllabic words where the syllable division is unclear, the phonetic division being ambiguous, and there being no stress or morphological grounds to help decide the matter, as in *table, pudding, open, extra, balloon,* and many more. Should these words be analysed as *pu-dding* or *pudd-ing,* etc.? Intuitions, it seems, vary enormously as to where the syllable boundary falls in such cases. To avoid the risk of an uncontrollable arbitrariness creeping into the profile procedure, therefore, we avoid making a decision as to whether these word-medial consonants are -C or C-. Instead, we recognise an indeterminate category, -C-, to which we assign all cases of this kind. -C- does not stand for 'medial consonant' (which would presuppose a word-based analysis) but for 'consonants whose distributional status is unclear, with respect to adjoining syllables'. These cases are listed in the two rightmost columns in the upper part of the chart. These columns are not as large as the others, reflecting the fact that in clinical samples these problem cases are relatively uncommon. The left-hand column (-C-) is used for single consonants; the right-hand column for consonant clusters (-CC(C)-), listed according to the *first* consonant in the cluster.

We can illustrate the way in which segments are assigned to different sections of the chart using the following examples:

cat	*cowboy*	*open*	*try*	*I*
[k æ t]	[k aʊ|b ɔɪ]	[əʊ p ə n]	[tr aɪ]	[aɪ]
C-V-C	C- V C- V	V -C V-C	CC V	V

running	*streams*	*destroy*	*invite*	
[r ʌ n|ɪ. ŋ]	[str i: mz]	[d ɪ str ɔɪ]	[ɪ nv aɪ t]	
C-V-C V -C	CCC-V-CC	C-V-CCC- V	V -CC-V-C	
		(-CCC- placed	(-CC- placed	
		along the *s* line)	along the *n* line)	

3.6 The classification in terms of sound types is made on conventional phonetic lines, bearing in mind those phonetic distinctions that are important in the English sound system.

3.6.1 Consonants are grouped vertically in terms of place and manner of articulation, viz.

Plosives
Affricates } front consonants being placed
Fricatives } higher up the chart than
Nasals } back consonants, within each
Approximants } category

For the first three categories, for initial and final consonants, voiceless consonants are placed on the left, and voiced consonants on the right. The layout is thus as follows:

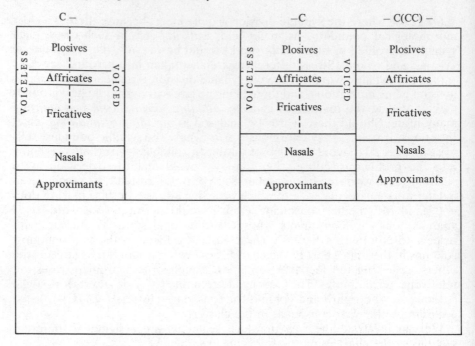

3.6.2 The following phone-types are recognized within these consonant categories:

plosives	p b t d k g	initially, finally and 'unclear' (see 3.5.2)
affricates	tʃ dʒ	
fricatives	f v θ ð s z ʃ	initially, finally and 'unclear'
	ʒ	finally and 'unclear'
	h	initially and 'unclear'
nasals	m n	initially, finally and 'unclear'
	ŋ	finally and 'unclear'
	m̩ n̩	finally
approximants	l r	initially, finally and 'unclear' (a slot for final [-r] is included, in view of the frequency of this item in regional speech)
	w j	initially and 'unclear'
	l̩	finally

3.6.3 Vowels are classified according to place and type of articulation:

short	ɪ	e	æ	ə	ʊ	ʌ	ɒ
long	iː	ɑː	ɜː	uː	ɔː		
diphthongs	eɪ	aɪ	ɔɪ	əʊ	aʊ	ɪə	ɛə ʊə
triphthongs	eɪə	aɪə	ɔɪə	əʊə	aʊə		

Within each category, close (or high) articulations are placed higher up the chart than open (or low) articulations; for short and long vowels, relatively front articulations are placed in the left-hand column, and relatively back articulations are placed in the right-hand column. Diphthongs and triphthongs are classified in terms of their direction of movement—towards [ɪ], [ʊ] or [ə].

At the bottom of the vowel column are placed those monosyllabic words in English which consist purely of a vowel. We regularly encounter Ps whose ability to use some of these words is different from the way in which they use vowels in CVC contexts, and we therefore classify them separately, in the first instance. The following items are involved:

[ə]	for unstressed *a, are, her, of, I*
[æ]	for stressed *a*
[ɪ]	for unstressed *he*
[ʊ]	for unstressed *who*
[i:]	for unstressed *he*
[ɑ:]	for *our*, and stressed *are* (in *r*-less accents)
[ɔ:]	for stressed *or* (in *r*-less accents)
[ɜ]	for unstressed *her* (in *r*-less accents)
[u:]	for unstressed *who*, and for *ooh*
[əʊ]	for *oh, O* (the letter)
[eɪ]	for stressed *a, A* (the letter)
[aɪ]	for stressed *I*
[iə]	for *ear* (in *r*-less accents)
[ɛə]	for *air* (in *r*-less accents)
[aʊɔ]	for stressed *our* (in *r*-less accents)

(Unstressed syllables consisting of consonant as well as vowel are profiled in the main section of the chart, in the usual way: see further, 3.8.)

We have not found it helpful to devote a separate section of the chart to the few cases where 'words' may consist of a single consonant, e.g. *m, sshh*. If one wishes to log these separately, there is a convenient blank box, adjacent to both [ʃ] and [m], in the initial consonant section.

Incorporating the above information into the sections described in 3.6 produces the layout on p. 66.

3.7* It will be recalled (from 3.3) that the accent reflected in this layout is RP. For Ps whose accents are a modified form of RP, it is possible to use this layout by making only minor modifications to the transcription. For example, if P's accent used an /əʊ/ diphthong where the initial element was further back, viz. [oʊ], it would be a simple matter to alter the relevant symbol on the chart (remembering to note the change under 'Accent Conventions' on the transcriptional page). Many of the more common regional variations can be handled in this way. But the systemic repercussions of changing one vowel value should be noted. In many accents, whole sets of changes would need to be incorporated, if an adequate account of P's phonological system were to emerge. Indeed, in an accent which was markedly different from RP, the vowel section of the chart would have to be replaced by an analysis more

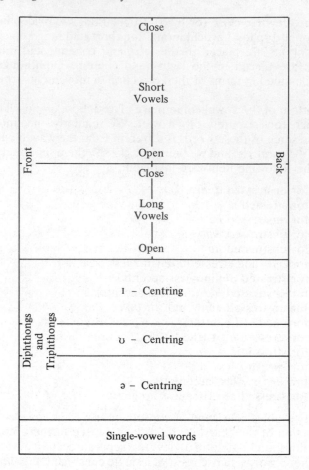

suited to that accent. (T would have had to do this anyway, of course, as part of his general evaluation of the dialect norms of an area, in relation to a decision concerning his therapeutic goals.) The present chart, therefore, must be used with caution: its organizational principles are of general application, but its descriptive categories (especially in the vowel section) must always be checked against the accent norms which identify T's teaching goals.

3.8 The distinction between stressed and unstressed syllables is also incorporated into the procedure, as P's abilities often vary in this respect. A horizontal line is therefore drawn within each phone-type for C-, V and -C. (Space constraints did not allow the extension of this convention to other sections of the chart.) The use of a phone in a *stressed* syllable is placed *above* this line. The use of a phone in an *unstressed* syllable is placed *below* this line. For example, in the word *singing,* as pronounced ['sɪŋɪŋ], the first [ɪ] and [ŋ] would be placed above the line, and the second below, as follows:

For syllabic consonants, the stressed/unstressed distinction does not apply. Also, for RP, the use of schwa [ə] is restricted to unstressed syllables, and therefore one would expect to find marks only in the lower section of that box on the chart. (In other accents, of course, where schwa may be used in stressed syllables, the upper section of the schwa box would be in use.)

When a stress pattern clearly motivates a syllabic division, we follow the stress, regardless of other (e.g. morphological) considerations. For example, one P said *taxi* as ['tæk — 'si:], which was accordingly profiled as two syllables, with a final [-k] and initial [s-].

3.9 The vertical lines which divide each box reflect the traditional distinctions in the study of articulatory disability. The first column refers to *correct* phones—that is, the target phone has been correctly articulated (as far as T can tell). The middle column refers to *omitted* phones, in relation to the target syllable. The third column refers to the *substituted* phones which T considers to be abnormal, in relation to the target phone. For example, we may take the following items, and see how they would be noted in relation to the [p] box in initial C- position (assuming a stressed syllable in each case):

target syllable	*pig* [pɪg]	*pig* [pɪg]	*pig* [pɪg]
P's pronunciations	[pɪg] [pi:]	[ɪg] [ɪ:]	[tɪg] [ʔɪ]

profiled as

For box 1: p— with 'll' marks in the correct column. For box 2: p— with 'll' marks in the omitted column. For box 3: p— with 't ı ʔ ı' marks in the substituted column.

Phone-tokens are added to the relevant part of each box, as they are encountered in the transcription. A typical box at the end of this process might look like this:

p— box: correct column (upper) has 'ʜɪ ı', omitted column (upper) has 'ı', substituted column (upper) has 't ı h ı / p w ı'; correct column (lower) has 'ııı', substituted column (lower) has 'h ı'.

This would mean: in the sample, P produced initial [p] correctly 6 times in stressed syllables and 3 times in unstressed syllables; he omitted the phone in a stressed syllable once; he replaced it in a stressed syllable by [t] once, by [h] once, and by a [pw] cluster once; and in an unstressed syllable by [h] once. Totalling up, of P's 15 initial [p-] targets, he was correct 9 times (see further, 3.20, for a discussion of quantitative summaries of the data).

3.10 Because -C- and -CC- represent phones whose syllabic status is uncertain (cf. 3.5.2), it is not possible to use the distinction between stressed and unstressed syllable systematically. The vertical columns explained in 3.9 do apply, however. So, for example, the pronunciation of the word *cabin* as ['kæbɪn] would involve a mark in the first column opposite [b]; ['kæɪn] would involve a mark in the second column; and, say, ['kækɪn] would require the [k] substitution to be noted in the third column. The (uncommon) cases of consonant clusters are written into the chart as they occur, using the first element in the cluster as the index for its position, e.g. in *sister*, the [-st-] cluster would be indicated as follows:

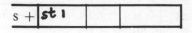

Correct, omitted or substituted forms would be assigned to the columns in the usual way.

3.11 The classification of consonant clusters is made in terms of (a) clusters containing two elements; and (b) clusters containing three or more elements. Initial and final clusters are presented across the bottom of the chart, using the first element of the cluster as the index. There is no space to make use of the stressed/unstressed distinction, but all clusters are classified in terms of correct/omitted/substituted phones. For a cluster to be placed in the *correct* column, the whole of the cluster must be correct; if only one element is correct, the form is placed in the *substitutions* column. If neither element is correct, the *substitutions* column is again used. A mark is placed in the *omissions* column only if the *whole* of the cluster is missing.

There are sufficiently few possibilities for 2-element clusters in English to permit the presentation of a complete list; likewise, for initial 3-element clusters. Final 3-element clusters, and the (less common) 4-element clusters, are too numerous to list conveniently, however; so this section of the chart is simply left blank, items being added in an ad hoc manner as they occur in the sample (which is not often).

The cluster inventory is therefore as follows:

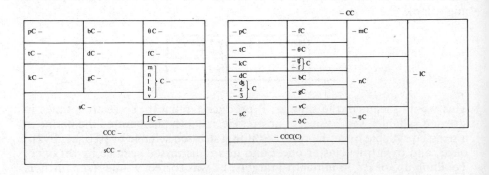

3.11.1 The assignment of clusters to this section of the chart can be illustrated from the following examples:

target pronunciation	*stop* [stɒp]	*stop* [stɒp]	*cats* [kæts]	*lump* [lʌmp]
P's pronunciation	[stɒp]	[tɒp]	[kæ]	[lʌb]

profiled as

s	p–				s	p–					–t	θ				–m p		b ı
	t–	ı				t–		t ı				s	ı			d		
	k–					k–										f		

A complete line, taken from a recent profile, was as follows:

t	r–	ı		tw ıɪɪ ʧ ɪɪɪ
	j–			
	w–			

This means that of 8 attempts at the [tr-] cluster in the sample, 1 was correct, there were no omissions, and there were 7 errors—in 4 cases, the cluster was replaced by [tw], and in 3 cases by [tʃ].

3.12* The model of analysis described above has been devised to handle connected speech as a series of isolated lexical and grammatical items. Thus a sentence such as *the dog is barking*, pronounced as [ðə 'dɒg ız 'bɑːkɪŋ], would be transcribed with each word on a separate line, somewhere on the transcription page; and each stressed and unstressed syllable would then be transferred onto the profile chart. In this case, seeing the sentence as a sequence of separate words poses no analytic problems. But if the sentence had been *the car is . . .* , pronounced [ðə 'kɑːr ız], there would be a problem, due to the occurrence of 'linking' *r*. If P's accent were RP, we would not wish to call this [r] a final consonant in the syllable, as it is not used when the syllable is spoken in isolation. The profile chart therefore has a separate section, where segmental modifications due to the connectivity of words in running speech can be located. This is the section marked *Conn.* in the bottom right-hand corner of the chart.

The procedure for using this section is as follows. The unaffected part of a syllable is profiled in the upper part of the chart, in the usual way. The segment(s) affected by the connected speech are *not* profiled in the same way, but are listed in the Conn. section as they occur. For example, if the sequence were *he can buy* . . . with *can* being pronounced [kəm], because of the influence of the following [b], the initial [k] and the vowel would be assigned to their appropriate places in the upper half of the chart; the final segment would be assigned to the Conn. section thus:

-n → -m /b-

(which reads: final [-n] was pronounced as [-m] in the context of a following [b-]). The linking *r* example above would be written thus:

CV → CVr /V-

(which reads: a syllable consisting of a consonant and a vowel was pronounced with a following [r] in the context of a following initial vowel). Of course, any convenient notation can be used, as long as it makes clear which segments have been affected, and the nature of the context in which the modification occurs.

When a segment has been *elided,* as part of normal connected speech, it is profiled in the usual way, e.g. *police* [pli:s] would be assigned to the [pl-] cluster box, and [ds] of *medicine* ['medsın] would be assigned to the -CC- column, and so on. Any general observation concerning P's use of casual or careful speech styles could be noted on the final supplementary page (under Variants). The only cases which might be placed under Conn. are those where the elision is such that there is no clear place for the item elsewhere on the chart, e.g. [f] in *cup of tea* ['kʌpf'ti:], [mn] in *how many times* ['haʊmnı 'taɪmz].

3.13 The remaining column on the profile summarizes the stress pattern in polysyllabic words in the sample. The three disyllabic patterns are listed (strong-weak, as in *Móndăy;* weak-strong, as in *tŏdáy;* and strong-strong, as in *téabág*). Longer sequences are written in as they occur, under the heading 3, e.g. *telephone* as ´ ˇ ´ . The number of correct instances of a target stress pattern is given in the left-hand column of this section; incorrect stress patterns are listed in the right-hand column. For example,

´ ˇ ⊔⊬ l	´ ´ lll
	´ l

would mean that of 10 ´ˇ patterns attempted, 6 were correct, 3 were produced as ´´ (e.g. ['mʌndeɪ] becoming ['mʌn'deɪ]) and 1 was produced as a single stressed syllable (e.g. ['mʌndeɪ] becoming ['mʌn]).

3.14 To illustrate the whole of the above procedure in operation, a short sample from a language-delayed child is given below, with the profiling decisions given alongside. The profile of the sample then follows on pp. 74–5. The accent is RP.

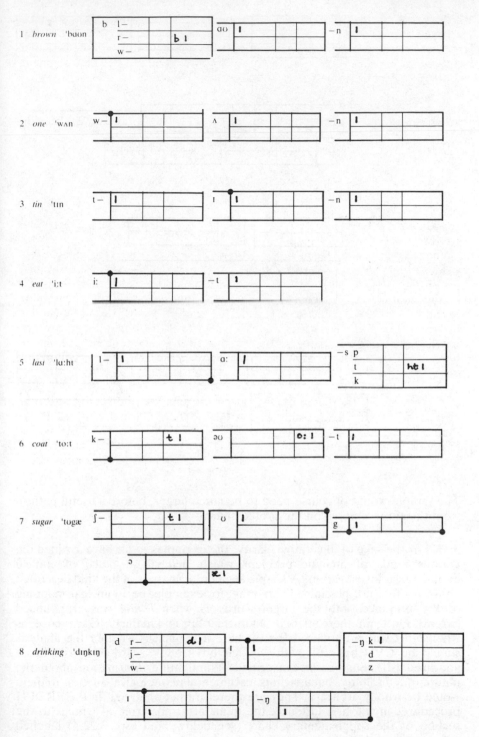

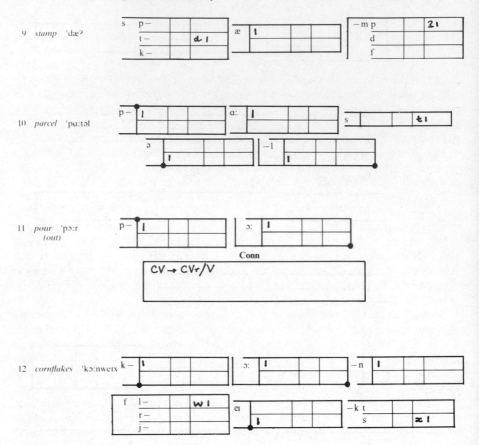

9   *stamp*   'dæʔ

10   *parcel*   'pɑːtəl

11   *pour*   'pɔːr
     (out)

Conn

CV → CVr/V

12   *cornflakes*   'kɔːnweɪx

The sample would of course need to be much larger, before a useful pattern would begin to emerge on the profile chart.

3.15 For the sake of illustrative clarity, the examples so far have avoided the various kinds of analytic problem which bedevil so much of clinical phonological investigation. A simple segmental analysis of the kind described above is often not possible. There may, for example, be an unclear mapping of P's utterance onto the target word, as when *lemon* was pronounced [woːnf]. Or again, there might be an unclear division in the CVC sequence, as when *bowl* was pronounced [boːʊ]: here it is unclear whether the analysis should be CV ([b] [oːʊ], with [-l] deleted) or CVC ([b] [oː] [-ʊ]—i.e. a vocalized [-l]). Such cases can provide illuminating information about the nature of a disability, but assigning a segmental phonological analysis to them would be wholly arbitrary. They are therefore not analysed, in the PROPH procedure, in the first instance: the items are transferred as wholes to the section of the supplementary chart (see below, and esp. 3.22.5) labelled *unanalysed*. Alternative methods of phonological analysis may then be tried out. The use of the *unanalysed* section is therefore recommended whenever there is any doubt concerning the assignment of segments on the profile chart.

3.16* Having completed the transcriptional page and the accompanying profile chart, and allowed for the existence of awkward cases, the PROPH procedure is in a sense complete. Certainly, the discipline of carrying out the transcription, and of analysing it systematically, can be sufficient to develop a good grasp of P's main problems. And because the profile chart provides a comprehensive frame of reference for segment distribution and phonetic type, it is a straightforward matter to identify some of the gaps, imbalances, and so on. We would therefore expect many Ts to find the exercise so far a sufficient basis for principled therapy. But if one wants to make a more formal statement concerning the nature of P's disability, or to evaluate the effects of therapy, some kind of qualitative or quantitative analysis is required. In many cases, in fact, we have found that a systematic analysis of the PROPH description brings to light patterns in the data that were not intuitively obvious from an impressionistic scrutiny of the profile chart. Sometimes, indeed, a further analysis is the only way to proceed, when the profile presents ambiguous or conflicting patterns.

There is a second reason why further analysis is desirable. The segmental description carried out above is only one way of handling phonological data. There are other ways of doing phonology which would make different assumptions about the data, and which might lead to alternative hypotheses about the nature of the disability. It is in our view essential to build aspects of these alternative analyses into a clinical procedure, to avoid being blinkered by the constraints of one's favourite model. It is not practicable to incorporate everything into a single procedure, nor is there a point in analysing the whole of one's sample systematically from three or four theoretical points of view. As long as the crucial theoretical insights of the various approaches are borne in mind, the dangers of narrow vision can be minimized. But for this to happen, specific guidelines need to be built into the procedure.

There are thus these two positive reasons why we have found it helpful to construct an analytic section to the PROPH procedure, and this has been printed on a separate set of three pages. There is also an important negative reason. It will be apparent that, from the viewpoint of an ideal profile procedure (cf. 1.10.2), PROPH is lacking an important dimension: it contains no acquisitional information. However, the fact of the matter is that recent studies of phonological acquisition have shown very clearly that the order of emergence of the sound segments of English is much more difficult to state than had previously been supposed. The traditional view, that it is possible to talk in terms of a certain sound being acquired first, or a certain set of sounds being acquired by 2, 2½ etc., has been shown to involve serious oversimplification, ignoring such matters as the way lexical variation affects the acquisition of a sound, the nature of the phonological learning processes which affect more than single segments, and the range of individual differences between children. It is therefore not possible, as yet, to construct a profile chart in which [m], say, was singled out as an early-learned segment, [ʃ] as a late-learned segment, and so on. For this kind of statement to be useful, it would

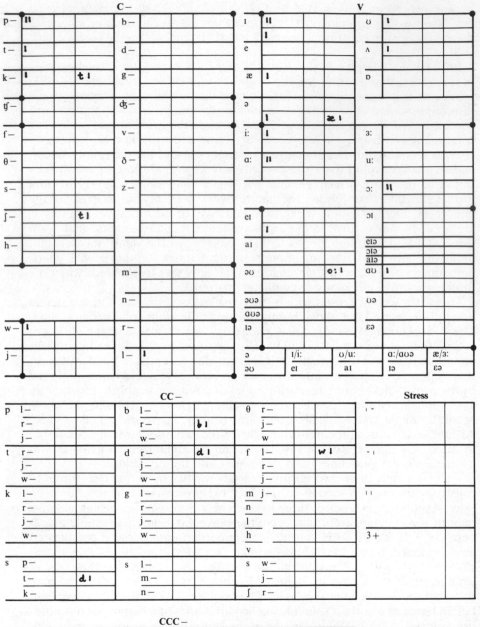

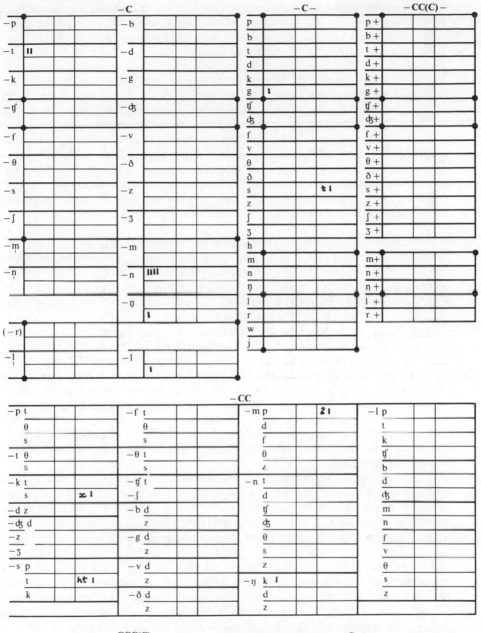

have to make clear whether one was talking about production or perception of the segment, in what kind of phonological context, in what range of words—and sufficient empirical research has not been done to make this possible. We have therefore avoided an acquisitional statement in the PROPH procedure. We have no objection to Ts using some typographical means to highlight certain segments on the chart, if their experience leads them to expect that early teaching would be fruitful; but this is a long way from the research-based synthesis of findings which would enable a developmental scale to be used with confidence as the basis of a remediation procedure.

Lacking an acquisitional perspective, the main reasoning which is used in carrying out phonological assessment and remediation is based on a consideration of the articulatory phonetic parameters and contrasts involved, in relation to what is known about the frequency and distribution of sounds in English. Here, a standard set of procedures for working through the profile data has been found to be helpful.

3.17 In view of the complex appearance of the supplementary pages, the first point to be stressed is that in routine clinical use, only *parts* of the procedure need to be referred to, for any one patient. It has been rare, in our experience, to need to analyse the sample from all the points of view represented on these pages. What must be appreciated, of course, is the kinds of information which these pages make available.

Essentially, each 'box' on the supplementary pages contains a numerical summary of some aspect of the data contained in the profile chart. For example, one might want to know what proportion of sounds P uses correctly in initial position compared with final position; what proportion of errors are due to problems of voicing, as opposed to other types of problem; whether a certain sound is replaced more frequently by one type of sound than another; and so on. To obtain the required information, it is necessary to work systematically through the profile chart, counting the instances of a phenomenon; the result is then transferred to the relevant box on the supplementary pages.

There are of course hundreds of possible ways of scanning the profile data in the hope of discovering interesting patterns. On the supplementary pages, we have given only those procedures which we have found to be particularly useful in carrying out assessments and remediation. Ts may have other scanning procedures which they might wish to add.

3.17.1 In scanning a profile chart, it is easy to lose one's place unless a disciplined method is used. If one is looking for, say, examples of voiceless phones being used as substitutions, one might start with C-, and move on to -C and then -C-, working horizontally first and then downwards. Alternatively, one might try to do all C- first, starting with [p] and [b] and working downwards, and then later moving to the -C column. It does not matter which procedure one adopts, as long as one adopts *some* procedure. Before we learned this lesson, we wasted a great deal of time by commencing to scan the chart for a feature, having to stop to cope with some distraction, and then continuing with the scan along a completely different path from where we had stopped—with the result that some boxes on the chart were scanned twice, and some not at all!

3.18 There are four main kinds of information presented on the supplementary pages:

(a) an inventory of the phones used in the data;
(b) a classification of the phones P uses, in relation to adult language targets;
(c) a statement of notable phonological features and processes in the data;
(d) a section in which further observations about the segmental phonological analysis can be made.

These kinds of information are laid out as follows:

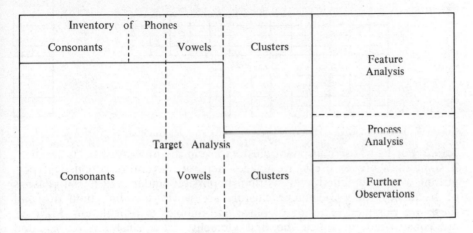

3.19 The inventory of phones is made regardless of the target words which P may have been aiming at. Each phone represented in the transcription is counted and classified, in terms of place and manner of articulation (for consonants) and in relation to the cardinal vowel diagram (for vowels). The phones involved in consonant clusters are included here, with additional information about clusters given below: 3.19.2).

This section of the procedure is not particularly helpful if there is little phonetic variability in the data, or if P's targets are quite clear. Under such circumstances, it would be more fruitful to proceed to a target analysis directly (see 3.20). But for data which is difficult to interpret (as in much dyspraxic speech), where targets are unclear and phonetic variability is considerable, there is little else once can do other than make a simple inventory of phones. One can at least establish, in this way, whether P is focussing on a particular place or manner of sound production, or avoiding certain areas of articulation.

3.19.1 Consonant phones are classified in terms of place and manner of articulation, with reference to their occurrence as singleton phones or as clusters. The distributional information is arranged vertically:

C refers to a singleton phone;
CC refers to a phone when it is the initial element in a cluster;
CC refers to a phone when it is the final element in a cluster.

The phonetic information is arranged horizontally:

> *Place of articulation:* bilabial; labio-dental; dental; alveolar; post-alveolar; retroflex; palato-alveolar; palatal; velar; uvular; pharyngeal; glottal; Other.
> *Manner of articulation:* plosive; affricate; fricative; nasal; approximant; Other pulmonic; Other non-pulmonic.

The two boxes therefore appear as follows:

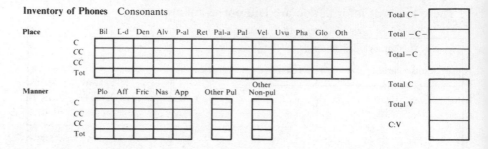

3.19.2 For Ps whose consonant clusters are in the process of being learned, it sometimes proves useful to make a separate inventory of clusters, permitting a more detailed analysis than is possible under 3.19.1. For reasons of frequency, only 2-element clusters are worth spending time on, and these are classified in terms of place and manner of articulation. Matrices are constructed, in which the first element of the cluster is represented vertically, and the second element horizontally. The small range of phonetic categories recognized has no theoretical significance: they are simply the categories which have turned up most commonly in samples. (Their approximation to the descriptive categories used in the target analysis is doubtless due to the fact that, when Ps are at the stage of cluster learning, their singleton consonants are usually well established. Errors in clusters commonly reflect articulations found elsewhere in the sound system of the language.)

The two boxes appear as follows, in the upper right of the second supplementary page:

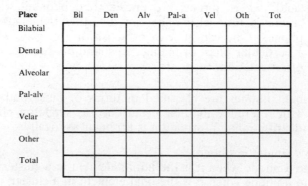

Manner	Plo	Aff	Fric	Nas	App	Oth	Tot
Plosive							
Affricate							
Fricative							
Nasal							
Approx							
Other							
Total							

3.19.3 The inventory of vowels is made by transferring the vowel values recognised in the transcription onto a cardinal vowel diagram. If the vowel in the transcription lacks a diacritic, it is assumed that the normal phonetic value for this vowel in RP obtains. For example, if there were 12 correct instances of [e] in the data, these would be placed on the CV diagram in the front mid position, as recommended by Gimson, and others. Diphthongs, etc. would be drawn in along conventional lines, with an accompanying indication of the number of instances. These examples are illustrated as follows:

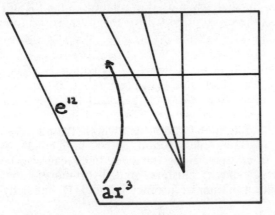

This would mean that, in the data, P used 12 [e] phones and 3 [aɪ] phones.

Incorrect vowel values for RP would have been identified in the transcription using cardinal vowel symbols (with diacritics, where necessary). These too are transferred to the diagram, and conflated with the correct phones, if any. For example, a pronunciation of *cat* as [ket] would have its [e] vowel counted along with any other [e] phones in the data.

The same principle applies whatever accent is being profiled: the vowel values are transferred onto the diagram using whatever information is known about the correct phonetic range for the units recognized in the transcription. For example, if a Cockney pronunciation of *day* had been recorded, as [daɪ], the relatively back starting-point of the [a] element in this diphthong would be shown in the line drawn on the CV diagram.

A complete vowel inventory for one P sample is given in the profile chart in 3.23.

3.19.4 It is sometimes helpful to have an overall indication of the number of phones transferred onto the profile chart (though in the present state of the art, such a total has little normative significance). A box is therefore provided in which can be placed:

(a) the total number of consonant phones (whether as singletons, or as part of clusters);
(b) the total number of vowel phones (whether 'pure' vowels or diphthongs);
(c) the consonant-vowel ratio (obtained by dividing (a) by (b)).

For example:

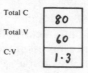

Total C	**80**
Total V	**60**
C:V	**1·3**

(a very low ratio, incidentally, suggestive of an open-syllable bias in the data).

Similarly, it is sometimes helpful to have an overall indication of the number of phones used initially, finally and 'medially' (bearing in mind the special sense of 'medial' when used in relation to the PROPH procedure: cf. 3.5.2). A box is therefore provided for this purpose, as follows:

Total C–	**126**
Total –C–	**12**
Total –C	**34**

This would mean that, in the sample as a whole, P used 126 consonant phones in initial position, 34 in final position, and 12 in 'medial' position.

A summary of clusters, along the same lines, can also be helpful. In the following box, 2-element clusters, and 3-(or more)-element clusters are totalled, in relation to their occurrence initially (I), 'medially' (M) and finally (F):

	I	M	F
CC	**1**	**-**	**8**
CCC(C)	**-**	**-**	**-**

This P had no clusters of 3 or more elements, had a single example of an initial 2-element cluster and 8 final 2-element clusters (an expected developmental bias, incidentally).

3.20 The second main type of information on the supplementary pages is a *target analysis* of the phones on the profile chart. Each of P's words on the transcriptional page is viewed in relation to the normal adult form for that word in P's speech community. If P's phones correspond to those of the target word, there is little more to be said, other than to count the number of correct occurrences in relation to their phonetic type. If P's phones do not correspond to those of the target, a detailed analysis is carried out of the errors made— whether omissions or substitutions, and if the latter, what kind of substitution. Singleton consonants, consonant clusters and vowels are each categorized in this way.

3.20.1 Target analysis of singleton consonants is made in terms of place and manner of articulation. First, a general statement is made of the total (T) number of correct (+) omitted (−) and substituted (Ø) phones, for each position in syllable structure (C-, -C-, -C). The matrix for place of articulation is as follows:

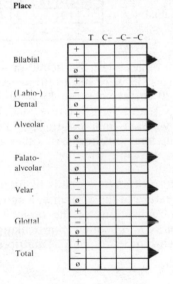

The matrix for manner of articulation is as follows:

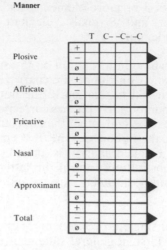

Manner

	T	C-	-C-	-C
Plosive +				
−				
ø				
Affricate +				
−				
ø				
Fricative +				
−				
ø				
Nasal +				
−				
ø				
Approximant +				
−				
ø				
Total +				
−				
ø				

Thus, for example, the following array of figures occurred in one sample:

Bilabial	T	C-	-C-	-C
+	20	13	1	6
−	19	–	3	16
ø	2	–	–	2

This meant that P had a target bilabial articulation 41 times in the sample; of these, 20 were correct (+), 19 were substitution errors (−), and there were 2 omissions (∅). Of the 20 correct phones, 13 were in initial position (C-), 6 were in final position (-C), and there was one 'medial' use of the phone (-C-). Of the 19 errors, 16 were in final position, and 3 were 'medial'. The 2 omissions were both in final position. All other boxes in the above two matrices are handled in the same way.

3.20.2 As it is the pattern of error which is likely to yield the most relevant information about the nature of the disability, à more detailed analysis is next made of the incorrect realizations of the target phones. Again, separate matrices are used for place and manner of articulation. The relevant parts of the summary matrices and the error analysis matrices are linked by arrows, as follows:

Target Analysis (Phones)   Error Analysis Realizations

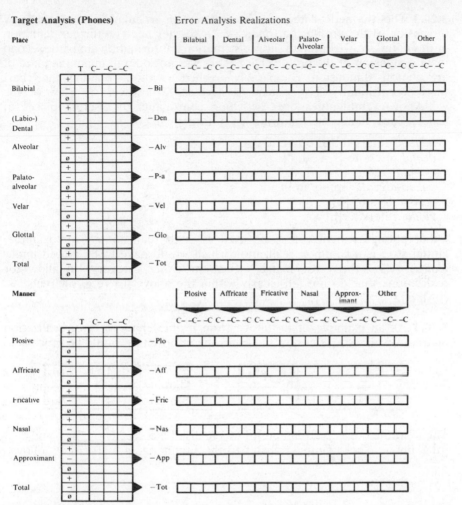

Using one of the lines of the place matrix as an example, one P sample produced the following results:

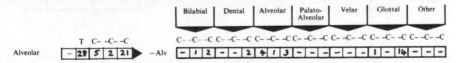

This meant that, of 28 incorrect realizations of alveolar targets,

3 were bilabials (1 'medial', 2 final),
2 were dentals (both final),
8 were alveolars (4 initial, 1 'medial', 3 final),
0 were palato-alveolar or velar,
15 were glottal (1 initial, 14 final),
there were no Other incorrect place realizations.

3.20.3 The phonetic categories of manner of articulation are a primary dimension of the profile chart (see 3.6.2), so they need no further definition at this point. As we opted to show distributional information along the second main dimension of the profile chart, there was no room to make the place of articulation dimension comparably explicit (without making the chart three-dimensional!). Explicitness is necessary, however, in view of the well-known ambiguities over assigning consonants to discrete places of articulation—hence the following list of target categories:

bilabial refers to [p, b, w, m]
dental refers to [f, v, θ, ð]
alveolar refers to [t, d, n, l, s, z, r]
palato-alveolar refers to [tʃ, ʤ, ʃ, ʒ, j]
velar refers to [k, g, ŋ]
glottal refers to [h]

Other phones will of course be used as error realizations—for example, glottal stop is a common realization which would have to be placed under *glottal*. Also, the error matrix needs an *Other* category, to allow for realizations that do not fall clearly within the above list (e.g. pharyngeals, clusters).

3.20.4 As an example of the move from profile chart to error realization matrix, we may consider how the following information would be processed:

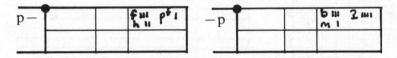

These profile boxes read: initial [p] was realised incorrectly 6 times, and final [p] 8 times. These figures transfer to the summarizing matrices as follows:

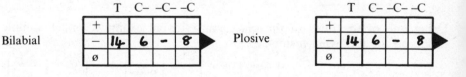

(In a real sample, of course, the figures in the two matrices would not be identical, because there would be further bilabial or plosive errors arising out of the incorrect realizations of other target phones in the data.) Of the initial errors, the *bilabial* target was realized as a bilabial once [pᶠ], a dental 3 times [f], and a glottal twice [h]; the *plosive* target was realized as an affricate once [pᶠ] and as a fricative 5 times [f, h]. Of the final errors, the *bilabial* target was realized as a bilabial 4 times [b, m] and as a glottal 4 times [ʔ]; the *plosive* target was realized as a plosive 7 times [b, ʔ] and as a nasal once [m]. This is summarized in the following way:

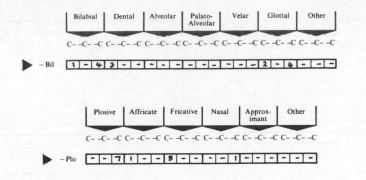

The use of a dash, or other symbol, to identify cells in the matrix where no data is recorded, is a procedure we recommend, as a means of checking that all formal possibilities have been considered.

3.20.5 The target analysis of clusters proceeds along similar lines. However, because of the extra element involved in a cluster, the matrices have a slightly different form, representing the articulatory sequences that form the clusters in English. From the *place* point of view, a cluster such as [-mp] can be seen as *bilabial + bilabial;* from the *manner* point of view, it is *nasal + plosive.* Before presenting the matrices on the chart, it will be convenient to show all possible 2-element initial and final sequences in terms of place and manner of articulation:

PLACE	Bil	Den	Alv	Pal-alv	Vel
Bilabial	-mp	-pθ -mf -mθ	pl- bl- pr- br- -pt -ps -bd -bz -md -mz	pj- bj- mj-	
Dental	θw-	-fθ	θr- fr- fl- -ft -fs -θt -θs -vd -vz -ðd -ðz	θj- fj- vj-	
Alveolar	tw- dw- sp- sm- sw- -sp -lp -lb -lm	-tθ -nθ -lf -lv -lθ	tr- dr- st- sl- sn- -lt -ld -ln -ts -dz -ls -ls -st -zd -nt -nd -ns -nz	tj- dj- nj- lj- sj- -ntʃ -ndʒ -ltʃ -ldʒ	sk- -sk -lk
Palato-alveolar			ʃr- -tʃt -dʒd -ʃt -ʒd		

PLACE	Bil	Den	Alv	Pal-alv	Vel
Velar	kw- gw-		kl- gl- kr- gr- -kt -ks -gd -gz -ŋd -ŋz	kj- gj-	-ŋk
Glottal				hj-	

MANNER	Plo	Aff	Fric	Nas	App
Plosive	-pt -kt -bd -gd		-pθ -ps -tθ -ts -ks -dz -bz -gz		pl- pr- pj- tr- tj- tw- bl- br- bw- dr- dj- dw- kl- kr- kj- kw- gl- gr- gj- gw-
Affricate	-tʃt -dʒd				
Fricative	sp- st- sk- -zd -ʒd -sp -st -sk -ft -θt -ʃt -vd -vð		-fθ -fs -θs -vz -ðz	sm- sn-	sl- fl- θr- fr- ʃr- θj- fj- hj- sj- vj- θw- sw-
Nasal	-mp -md -nt -nd -ŋk -ŋd	-ntʃ -ndʒ	-mf -mθ -mz -nθ -ns -nz -ŋz		mj- nj-
Approximant	-lp -lt -lk -lb -ld	-ltʃ -ldʒ	-lf -lv -lθ -ls -lz	-lm -ln	lj-

All 2-element clusters in the data are then assigned to the appropriate cell of these matrices, in terms of whether the cluster is a correct realisation of the target (+) or incorrect (−). (No further analysis of the incorrect cases is carried out at this point.) The summarizing diagrams, on the second supplementary page, are shown on p. 87 (the shaded cells are those where there are no 2-element target clusters in English).

Because of their frequency, it was not felt worthwhile to construct a matrix to handle more complex clusters in English. We prefer to list these as they occur, in the space above the 2-element matrices. Of course, if 3-element clusters were a particular focus of remedial attention, this ad hoc procedure would not suffice, and a systematic classification would have to be made.

There was space to provide only a general summary of the other patterns of error which characterize consonant clusters, and this is given in a separate

Place	Bil		Den		Alv		Pal-a		Vel		Oth	Total	
	+	−	+	−	+	−	+	−	+	−	−	+	−
Bilabial													
Dental													
Alveolar													
Pal-alv													
Velar													
Glottal													
Total													

Manner	Plo		Aff		Fric		Nas		App		Oth	Total	
	+	−	+	−	+	−	+	−	+	−	−	+	−
Plosive													
Affricate													
Fricative													
Nasal													
Approx													
Total													

matrix, located immediately under the heading *Target Analysis (Clusters)*. The vertical columns refer to the occurrence of a target cluster in initial (I), 'medial' (M) or final (F) syllabic positions. The horizontal lines refer to the main processes affecting the realization of the target:

CC(CC)	the cluster (2, 3 or 4 elements) has all its elements realized (though not necessarily in their correct phonetic form);
$C \rightarrow CC$	a target singleton consonant has been realized as a cluster;
$CC \rightarrow +V$	a target cluster has been realized with an intervening vowel;
$C_1C_2 \rightarrow C_1$	a 2-element cluster is reduced to its first element;
$C_1C_2 \rightarrow C_2$	a 2-element cluster is reduced to its second element;
$C_1C_2 \rightarrow C_3$	a 2-element cluster is reduced to a single element which is not phonetically identical with either C_1 or C_2.

These possibilities are summarized as follows:

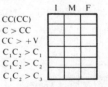

Other possibilities (e.g. $C_1C_2 \rightarrow C_3C_4$, $C_1C_2 \rightarrow VC_2$) can be listed in the adjacent space, if they occur.

3.20.6 As an example of the profiling procedure in relation to the 2-element consonant cluster matrices, the following words as pronounced by one child are analysed, with just the information about cluster production being transferred to the appropriate cell:

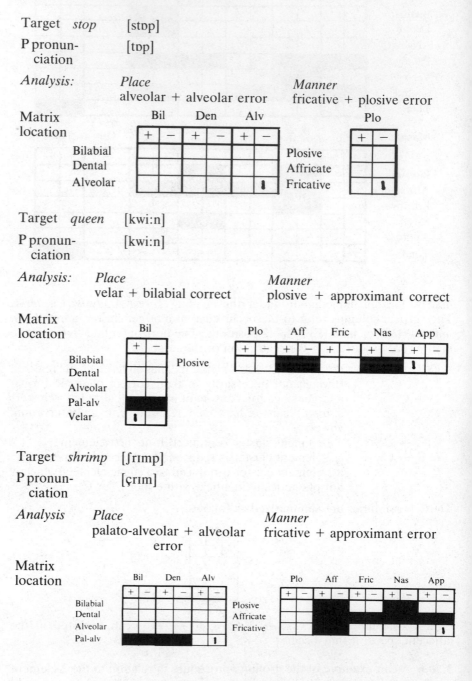

Target *stop* [stɒp]

P pronun- [tɒp]
  ciation

Analysis: *Place*
alveolar + alveolar error

Manner
fricative + plosive error

Target *queen* [kwi:n]

P pronun- [kwi:n]
  ciation

Analysis: *Place*
velar + bilabial correct

Manner
plosive + approximant correct

Target *shrimp* [ʃrɪmp]

P pronun- [çrɪm]
  ciation

Analysis *Place*
palato-alveolar + alveolar error

Manner
fricative + approximant error

These three words would have been transferred to the remaining cluster matrix in the following way:

stop [tɒp]   initial cluster reduced to second element

$$C_1C_2 > C_2 \quad \begin{array}{|c|c|c|} \hline \text{I} & \text{M} & \text{F} \\ \hline \textbf{I} & & \\ \hline \end{array}$$

queen [kwi:n]   initial cluster has both elements retained

$$CC(CC) \quad \begin{array}{|c|c|c|} \hline \text{I} & \text{M} & \text{F} \\ \hline \textbf{I} & & \\ \hline \end{array}$$

shrimp [çrɪm]   initial cluster has both elements retained (NB the error is not noted at this point, but on the place/manner matrices above)

$$CC(CC) \quad \begin{array}{|c|c|c|} \hline \text{I} & \text{M} & \text{F} \\ \hline \textbf{I} & & \\ \hline \end{array}$$

final cluster reduced to first element

$$C_1C_2 > C_1 \quad \begin{array}{|c|c|c|} \hline \text{I} & \text{M} & \text{F} \\ \hline & & \textbf{I} \\ \hline \end{array}$$

3.20.7 Target vowels are analysed along similar lines to singleton consonants. First, a general statement is made of the total number of correct (+) and incorrect (−) pure vowels, classified in terms of place of articulation. The two conventional cardinal vowel dimensions are used for this purpose, three divisions being recognized along each dimension, as follows (diphthongs are classified in terms of their initial element):

close (high)	[ɪ, ʊ, i:, u:, eɪ(ə), iə]
mid	[e, ə, ɜ:, ɔ:, ɔɪ(ə), əʊ(ə), ɛə, ʊə]
open (low)	[æ, ʌ, ɒ, ɑ:, aɪ(ə), aʊ(ə)]
front	[i:, e, æ, eɪ(ɔ), aɪ(ə), iə, ɛə]
central	[ɪ, ʊ, ə, ʌ, ɜ:, əʊ(ə), ʊə]
back	[u:, ɔ:, ɑ:, ɒ, ɔɪ(ə), aʊ(ə)]

The initial summaries are presented in the two small boxes in the upper left of the vowel column:

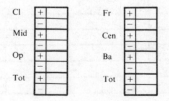

For example, P pronunciations of the target vowels in the following words would be analysed thus:

Target *bed* [bed]

P pronun-   [bæd]
ciation

Analysis: close-open   *front-back*
             mid error   front error

Location   Mid [matrix: + / − with mark in −]   Fr [matrix: + / − with mark in −]

Target   *cow* [kɑʊ]

P pronun-   [kɑʊ]
ciation

Analysis: close-open   *front-back*
             open correct   back correct

Location   Op [matrix: + with mark / −]   Ba [matrix: + with mark / −]

Vowel substitution errors may then be separately analysed, using the matrices adjoining the above. In the first matrix, each close, mid or open error is assigned to one of five cells, depending on whether the realization is *close, mid, open, unclear* (?) or *Other*. For example,

P [bɪd] for target [bi:d] illustrates a *close* error realization of a *close* target;
P [bed] for target [bi:d] illustrates a *mid* error realization of a *close* target;
P [bæd] for target [bi:d] illustrates an *open* error realization of a *close* target;
P [bëd] for target [bi:d] illustrates an *unclear* realization of a *close* target, as phonetically it fell midway between [ɪ] and [e];
P [bld] for target [bi:d] illustrates an *Other* realization of a close target.

The complete close-open matrix appears as follows:

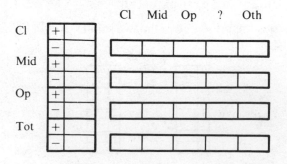

In this example, a data sample has been transferred to the matrix:

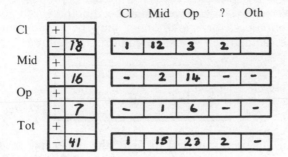

This pattern illustrates a marked tendency towards abnormally open articulations:

P makes 18 errors in his close vowel targets, of which 1 is realized as a close vowel, 12 are mid vowels, 3 are open vowels, 2 are Others;

P makes 16 errors in his mid vowel targets, of which 2 are mid vowels, 14 are open vowels;

P makes 7 errors in his open vowel targets, of which 1 is a mid vowel (contravening his general tendency) and 6 are open vowels.

Exactly the same analytic principles apply to the front-back matrix: each front, central or back error is assigned to one of five cells, depending on whether the realization is *front, central, back, unclear* (?) or *Other*. For example, P [bɒd] for target [bɪd] illustrates a *back* realisation of a *front* target; and so on. The complete front-back matrix appears as follows, along with some data which illustrates a marked tendency towards centralization, in the sample used:

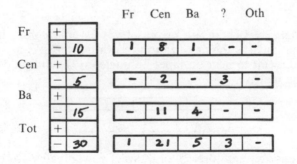

In particular, one should note:

P makes 10 errors in his front vowel targets, 8 of which are central;

P makes 11 errors in his back vowel targets, 11 of which are central.

3.20.8 While close-open and front-back errors provide a great deal of useful information about phonological disability, they by no means exhaust the patterns of vowel error encountered in P samples. In the rest of the vowel column, accordingly, we list the other error parameters which we have found it helpful to consider systematically:

(a) Vowel elements Pure vowels may be diphthongized (or triphthongized), and diphthongs (or triphthongs) may be monophthongized. The possibilities are summarized in a simple matrix, as follows:

	V	VV(V)	Other
V			
VV(V)			

Interpreting this diagram from left to right, the upper line reads:

1st cell: a target pure vowel is realized as a pure vowel;
2nd cell: a target pure vowel is realized as a diphthong or triphthong;
3rd cell: a target pure vowel is realized as something else (e.g. some kind of vocalized consonant, or an omission).

The lower line reads:

1st cell: a target diphthong or triphthong is realized as a pure vowel;
2nd cell: a target diphthong or triphthong is realized as a diphthong or triphthong;
3rd cell: a target diphthong or triphthong is realized as something else.

An example of a fairly primitive vowel pattern is as follows:

	V	VV(V)	Other
V	*12*	-	*1*
VV(V)	*23*	*1*	-

(b) Nasalization There are no nasal vowels in English, hence the only pattern to be noted is the nasalization of oral vowels. As nasal resonance is sometimes difficult to hear on tape, an unclear (?) cell is added, to produce the following matrix:

	Oral	Nasal	?
Oral			

The three cells are therefore: (i) oral target vowel realized as oral vowel; (ii) oral target vowel realized as nasal vowel; (iii) oral target vowel realized with unclear nasality.

(c) Stressing We have sometimes found it helpful to summarize the abnormal stressing of vowels, as when an unstressed target vowel is produced with a degree of stress, or a stressed target vowel produced without stress. Examples from Ps include *'kick'ing, 'bal'loon,* where an unstressed syllable has been stressed, with consequent change in the vowel quality of *bal* ([bə] becoming [bæ]); and *ele'phant* [ələ'fænt], where a target stressed vowel is

unstressed, and a target secondary stress (*fant*) has been made primary. The main possibilities are included on the following matrix:

	V́	V̆	?
V́			
V̆			

Here, the upper line reads (from left to right):

1st cell: a stressed target vowel is realized as a stressed vowel;
2nd cell: a stressed target vowel is realized as an unstressed vowel;
3rd cell: a stressed target vowel is realized with an unclear stress value.

The lower line reads (from left to right):

1st cell: an unstressed target vowel is realized as a stressed vowel;
2nd cell: an unstressed target vowel is realized as an unstressed vowel;
3rd cell: an unstressed target vowel is realized with an unclear stress value.

An example of a fairly common over-stressing pattern is as follows (taken from an adult P whose speech style, impressionistically, might be described as 'staccato' or 'word-at-a-time'):

	V́	V̆	?
V́	46	–	–
V̆	38	–	11

(d) Rounding Abnormal variations in the pattern of lip-rounding on pure vowels can be noted, using the following matrix. The first line reads (from left to right): a target rounded vowel may be realized as (i) rounded, (ii) unrounded, or (iii) with unclear rounding. The second line reads (from left to right): a target unrounded vowel may be realized as (i) rounded, (ii) unrounded, or (iii) with unclear rounding.

	Roun	Unr	?
Roun			
Unr			

The following example is from a sample of speech from a dysarthric P, whose lips were markedly affected, with unrounding a noticeable consequence:

	Roun	Unr	?
Roun	1	28	15
Unr	–	35	–

(e) Length   A common feature of phonological disability is abnormality in the length P gives to target pure vowels: short vowels become long, and long vowels become short. Sometimes, the length is indeterminate. These three main possibilities are summarized in the following matrix, whose upper line reads (from left to right): a target short vowel is realized as (i) a short vowel, (ii) a long vowel, or (iii) with uncertain length; in the lower line (reading again from left to right), a target long vowel is realized (i) by a short vowel, (ii) by a long vowel, or (iii) with uncertain length.

	V	V:	?
V			
V:			

A common source of unintelligibility in the connected speech of children with articulation problems lies in the way long vowels are shortened, often with concomitant alterations in quality. One such sample produced the following summary:

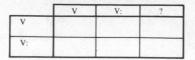

	V	V:	?
V	47	–	8
V:	31	3	11

3.21 Doubtless because of the nature of our initial training, we find ourselves more at home with an analysis in terms of phones and phonemes, and in any systematic investigation of phonological data, we always begin in this way. Indeed, an initial representation of a data sample in terms of phones seems unavoidable, whatever one's theoretical inclinations. However, there is also a great deal to be gained by carrying out an analysis in terms of distinctive features, phonological processes, or prosodies (in the sense of Firth). We have therefore given over a section of the supplementary pages to the analysis of the data using certain of the notions derived from these alternative theories.

3.21.1* The analysis of phonological disability in terms of phonetic feature contrasts can be illuminating, and indeed, there are many such features hidden in the terminology used earlier (bilabiality, plosiveness, etc.), though these are not conceived as sets of binary oppositions. The set of matrices on the top of the third supplementary page is available for data analysis in terms of binary oppositions, if required. We have often found the need to analyse our samples in terms of the contrast of *voicing,* so we have labelled the first matrix accordingly. The other matrices have been left blank, available for the analysis of other feature contrasts (such as grave v. acute, nasal v. oral, sharp v. plain).

For the voicing matrix, each consonant phone in the profile chart is analysed in terms of its voiced/voiceless relationship to its target. If the target phone is voiced, and P's realization is also voiced, the feature is said to be *maintained;* similarly, if the target phone is voiceless, and P's realization is also voiceless. On the other hand, if the target phone is voiced, and P's realization is voiceless, the feature is said to be *lost;* similarly if the target phone is voiceless, and P's realization is voiced. The only realization which does not fit into this system is glottal stop: if a target phone is replaced by a glottal stop, it would seem equally arbitrary to call it a voiced or a voiceless phone—we therefore avoid the decision, and classify [ʔ] substitutions separately, using the middle column of the matrix.

It is useful to know whether voicing contrasts are maintained or lost more frequently in initial, 'medial' or final position. These distinctions are thus incorporated under the two headings, as follows:

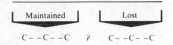

To make the voicing profile more discriminating, the above distinctions are related to the usual parameters of target place and manner of articulation, tabulated separately for ease of reading, as follows:

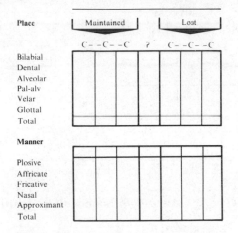

Transferring the information from a profile chart onto these matrices may be illustrated from the following examples.

Target *go* [gəʊ]   P's pronunciation [gəʊ]

Analysis: *Place*   C- velar
              Manner   C- plosive } voicing maintained

Matrix location

Target *cup* [kʌp]   P's pronunciation [tʌp]

Analysis: *Place*   C- velar   -C bilabial ⎫
              Manner   C- plosive -C plosive ⎬ voicing maintained, both cases
                                                 ⎭

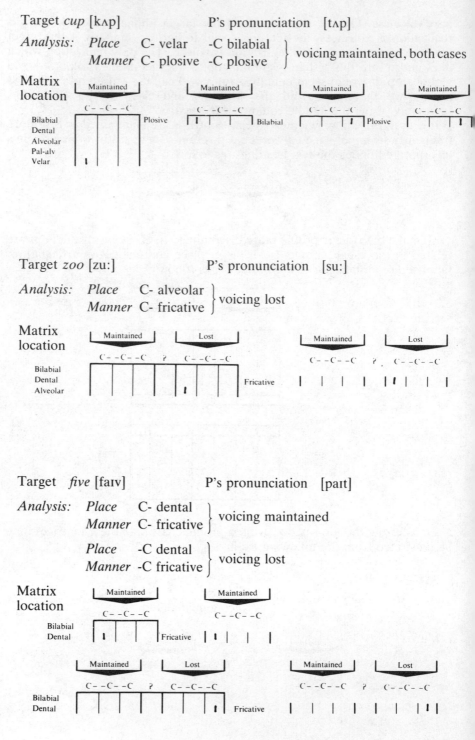

Target *zoo* [zu:]   P's pronunciation [su:]

Analysis: *Place*   C- alveolar ⎫
              Manner   C- fricative ⎬ voicing lost
                                       ⎭

Target *five* [faɪv]   P's pronunciation [paɪt]

Analysis: *Place*   C- dental   ⎫
              Manner   C- fricative ⎬ voicing maintained
                                       ⎭

              Place   -C dental   ⎫
              Manner   -C fricative ⎬ voicing lost
                                       ⎭

Target   *cut* [kʌt]   P's pronunciation   [kʌʔ]

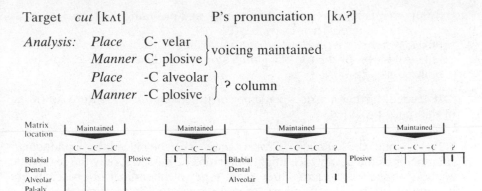

Analysis: Place   C- velar
              Manner   C- plosive } voicing maintained
              Place   -C alveolar
              Manner   -C plosive } ʔ column

Subclassification in terms of place and manner of articulation relates to the target phones, and not to P's realizations. A complete voicing analysis in terms of manner of articulation is given in the profile chart in 3.23.

3.21.2 Consonant clusters may also be given a feature analysis in terms of voicing (or any other feature), and we provide one matrix in which we illustrate our approach to this category. The 2-element clusters in English can be neatly grouped in terms of 3 types:

(a) both elements voiceless (including cases where the second element has been devoiced, under the influence of the first element), e.g. [pl̥-, pr̥-, pj̥-, tr̥-, tj̥-, tw̥, -pt, -pθ, -ps, tθ, ts];
(b) both elements voiced, e.g. [bl-, br-, bw-, dr-, dj-, -lv, -lz, -bd, -gd, -vd];
(c) mixed voicing (first element voiced, second voiceless), e.g. [-mp, -mf, -mθ, -nt, -ntʃ, -lp].

There are many possibilities of error. For example, the [bl-] cluster might be realized as:

[bl-]   i.e. voicing maintained,
[pl̥-]   i.e. voicing lost,
[pl-]   i.e. voicing partly lost,
[bl̥-]   i.e. voicing partly lost,
[b-]   i.e. voicing maintained (the cluster reduction being noted else-
        where, cf. 3.20.5),
[p-]   i.e. voicing lost,

and so on. In our summary, we recognize 3 main patterns of error, as follows:

Maintained, i.e. the voicing pattern in the cluster is maintained, regardless of which particular phones are used, e.g.
[bl-]   is realized as [bl-, br-, dr-, b-, gw-],
[-pt]   is realized as [-pt, -ft, -ks, -p],
[-mp]   is realized as [-mp, -mf, -nt].
Lost, i.e. the voicing pattern in the cluster is lost, regardless of which particular phones are used, e.g.
[bl-]   is realized as [pl-, pl̥-, bl̥-, p-, l̥-, s-],
[-pt]   is realized as [-bd, -bt, -v, -m, -a (!)],

[-mp]   is realized as [-md, -ɸp, -p, -m], and including the (rare) reversals ·
of voicing, such as [-m̩b, -fb].
Other, where it is unclear what the voicing pattern is, due to auditory
indeterminacy, or the use of a glottal stop within the cluster, e.g. [-pt] being
realized as [-ʔt, -ʔ].

If needed, further matrices could be constructed for other feature contrasts,
in the space provided.

3.21.3* Under the heading of *Process analysis* can be placed those phonological aspects of the data which might otherwise be missed if only the segmental
analysis above were used. Three main types of phonological processes are
identified, in this view, and we provide space to allow information to be
entered under each of the headings, though in practice certain of the headings
are more useful than others.

(a) Syllable structure processes are those where the structure or use of a
target syllable is altered in some way—usually by simplification. For example,
a word might have a syllable deleted, as when P says ['nɑ:nə] for *banana:*
these cases would be written in under *S. deletion.* A syllable might be added
to a word, in which case the entry would be made under *S. addition* (e.g. the
patterns of reduplication common in early speech, as in ['kaka] for *cat*). The
deletion of a consonant (in any position) would be handled under *C. deletion*
(e.g. [kɑ:] for *cat*), and the addition of a consonant under *C. addition* (e.g.
[bweɪv] for *wave*). Under *Other* would be placed any further syllable structure
processes, e.g. affecting vowels as opposed to consonants, or affecting
particular types of consonant cluster.

(b) Assimilations refer to the way in which consonants or vowels work in
combination within a word or phrase—one segment being influenced by
another, or whole sets of segments being affected by some more general
process. In a pronunciation of *dog* as [gɒg], for example, it is plain that the
final [-g] has influenced the pronunciation of the initial [d-]. To say that [d]
has been substituted by [g] would make little sense without referring to the [g]
elsewhere in the word. In the profile chart above, however, the only fact that
could be recorded is the [d]-[g] substitution. Hence, it is important to have an
additional section in the procedure in which these contextual influences can
be recorded, when the analyst notices them. (They are common, for example,
in samples of dyspraxic speech.)

Two types of assimilatory process are named: *C harmony* ('consonant
harmony'), whereby a consonant in one position within a word becomes more
like or identical with one from another position in the word, or in an adjacent
word. The *dog* example above is typical, showing the process of 'velar
assimilation' (i.e. the apical consonant 'becomes' velar, in the context of a
velar consonant). In *V harmony* ('vowel harmony'), it is the vowel in a word
which becomes more like or identical to one from another position in the
same or a nearby word, e.g. the pronunciation of *rabbit* as ['wawa], in which
the [ɪ] vowel has become [a], because of the influence of the first [a]. Other
types of assimilatory process are not labelled separately, e.g. when a
consonant devoices, due to the influence of a neighbouring voiceless
consonant, or because it is occurring in a certain position in a word—such

information could if needed be placed under the heading of *Other,* in this column.

(c) Substitution processes handle the same kind of data as that recorded in the substitution columns on the profile chart, but a direct attempt is made to state a generalization, and not to restrict the statement to what is happening to an individual phone. For example, if fricatives are replaced by stops, a process of *stopping* might be said to be taking place, e.g. *zoo* as [du:], *fat* as [pat]. As it is possible to work out such generalizations from the profile chart above, however, by using the relevant matrices in the supplementary pages, this type of phonological process does not usually add anything to the information already gained by these earlier means. We therefore do not provide any subheadings, preferring to leave these to be added by those who would wish to commence their analysis with this approach directly.

(d) A further box is provided for noting down any other processes which do not seem to fall under any of the above headings, or whose assignment to one or other of the headings is uncertain.

An example of this section of the chart follows. It has been filled in by an analyst whose preferences were to do the segmental analysis first, using process analysis in a supplementary way. He has made most use of the C and V harmony boxes, and noted several syllable structure features. (It is recognized that, for someone whose analytic preferences are to proceed with process analysis directly, this section of the chart would be wholly inadequate; for such people, it would be advisable to use one of the available process-based procedures.)

Process Analysis

Syllable Structure	Assimilations	Substitutions
S Deletion police [pi:t]	C Harmony ŋ→t/t̚- (31)(47)	
S Addition ball [bɔbɔ:l] down [dav'nə]	b→g/t̚- (69) k→t/tʃ- (100)	
C Deletion CC- → C- (12)(33)(42)	V Harmony ɒ→I/i:- (7)	
C Addition sleeping ['ti:ptɪŋ]		?
Other	Other	

A notational summary of the process involved is used, whenever this is clear (e.g. [k] became [t] in the context of a preceding [tʃ], in line 100 of the transcriptional page); cluster simplification occurred (CC- becoming C-) in lines 12, 33 and 42 of the transcriptional page). In many cases, it is easier simply to write out the lexical item along with its phonetic realization, leaving a more general statement until later (often, until after further data has been analysed).

It should be noted that information about processes is derived from a consideration of the items listed on the transcriptional page, and not from the profile chart directly. For example, if P says *play tennis* as ['peɪ 'pens], it seems likely that the reason for the realization of /t-/ as [p] is due to the influence of the preceding [p]. On the profile chart, however, the only information recorded would be the abnormal substitution of [p] for /t/ in the appropriate column. There is no space on the profile chart to record abnormal contextual influences. Hence, the data on the transcriptional page must always be considered from the process viewpoint, at some point in the investigation, and any factors of potential interest transferred directly to the Process section of the supplementary pages.

3.22 Lastly, on the supplementary pages, we look back over the whole range of analyses which have been carried out, and extract certain types of information which are likely to be particularly helpful in assessment and remediation.

3.22.1 *Functional load* refers to the range of targets for which P uses a phone, in the sample. For instance, the phone [t] turned up in the following words, in one sample:

as the realization of initial /t-/, e.g. [tu:];
as the realization of initial /d-/, e.g. [tʌ] for *duck;*
as the realization of initial /tr-/, e.g. [taɪ] for *try;*
as the realization of final /-t/, e.g. [kæt];
as the realization of final /-p/, e.g. [kʌt] for *cup;*

and so on. By systematically scrutinizing the profile chart, it is easy to see the range of contexts in which a certain phone is used; and it is this range which is summarized in the functional load section. A convenient notation might be as follows (for the above example):

[t] ← /t-, d-, tr-, -t, -p, . . ./

If necessary, a tally could be kept of the number of instances related to each of these realizations, using superscripts, e.g.

[t] ← /t-[6], d-[2], tr-[1], -t[5], -p[2], . . .]

This would read: [t] was used 6 times for initial /t-/, twice for initial /d-/, and so on. This knowledge of the range of functions which [t] is called upon to perform, for this P, is an important element in T's decision about the severity of the disorder and its remediation.

3.22.2 *Variants* involves one looking at the items on the transcriptional page, and noting any cases where there is vacillation in P's production between two or more phones in relation to a particular target. For example, one P sometimes said [æ] for words containing a target /æ/, and sometimes said [e], e.g. repeated attempts at the word *man* produced [mæn, mæn, men, men, mæn]. Other [æ]/[e] alternations were observed elsewhere in the sample. [æ]/[e] would therefore be noted under *variants* on the final supplementary page—perhaps with a cross-reference to the relevant line numbers on the transcriptional page.

Another example of a set of variants was a P who sometimes replaced final plosives with a glottal stop, sometimes omitted them (zero, symbolised as ∅), and sometimes produced them reasonably well. Under variants, in this case, were notations such as [-p/-ʔ/-∅], [-t/-ʔ/-∅/-k], along with an indication of the target—/-p/, in the first case, /-t/ in the second.

This information is basically the reverse of that given under 3.22.1. Under *variants,* we are looking at any particularly important patterns of phonetic variability which expound a phonological target; under *functional load* we are looking at the range of phonological targets which a particular phonetic unit expounds.

3.22.3 Under the heading of *contrasts,* the aim is to note any sets of phones, conventionally seen as contrasting in phonetic terms, which the data shows to be wholly accurately maintained by P (100%+) or not accurately maintained at all (100%−). Take the following sample of data for initial plosives:

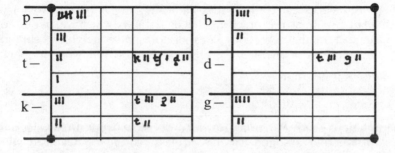

Here, the phonetic contrast between voiced and voiceless bilabial plosive is apparently able to be maintained: there are no confusions, and the postulate would be that the contrast is 100 per cent satisfactory (for this sample of data). Similarly, the contrast between bilabial and velar voiced plosives seems 100 per cent satisfactory. On the other hand, the contrast between alveolar voiced and voiceless plosives is 100 per cent unsatisfactory: /d-/ is sometimes realized as [t], and /t-/ is sometimes realized as [d]—apart from the other substitutions which affect these targets. The situation between /k-/ and /g-/ is a little more complex, due to the substitutions for /k-/; but it looks on the surface as if a contrast is being maintained. The situation between /t-/ and /k-/ is more complex still: here, the profile is ambiguous, suggesting that there is a possible contrast here (with several correct instances of both), but that it is often lost (with no less than 5 substitutions of [t] for /k-/).

Under the headings of 100%+ and 100%−, we note only those cases where the phonetic contrast seems clearly maintained, from the sample before us, or clearly lost. Such cases will provide essential focal points for remediation. An apparently stable contrast will provide a foundation for the teaching of less stable units. A wholly unstable contrast will suggest itself as an urgent candidate for remedial work. In *all* cases, of course, it would be important to check on the reliability of the data contained in the sample, and of the notion of contrast used above, by doing some structured work directly (such as auditory discrimination tasks).

The contrasts are briefly summarized under the respective headings, as follows (for the above example):

100%+   p-/b-, b-/g-, ?k-/g-
100%−   t-/d-

3.22.4 Under the heading of *indeterminacy* is noted any cases of regular uncertainty in carrying out the phonetic transcription of the data. It is a fact of clinical phonetic life that aspects of the data are going to be unclear—for whatever reason (poor recording, intrusive noise, P indistinct, T's ear). We have already used the set of indeterminate symbols to mark in the transcription these cases of uncertainty (cf. 3.3). Now, on the final page, any *regularly* occurring indeterminacies are given separate mention. For example, many items on the transcriptional page might have contained consonants whose voicing was a matter of doubt; or there may have been uncertainty concerning the degree of centralization of certain vowels. It is no service to the analysis to pretend that the data is clear, and to opt for one analysis over another, in such cases. Rather, it is clinically very important to let one's uncertainty be seen, as it is precisely this uncertainty which will in due course be a focus of remedial attention. We therefore find it helpful to summarize the more commonly occurring uncertainties, as in the following sample lines:

C   t/d/d̪, s/ʃ/ʂ/h, n/m/ṽ
V   e/ę/ë
Syll   ən/n̩

These notations read: our transcriptional decisions were often uncertain in respect of whether a sound was a voiceless, voiced or devoiced alveolar plosive; an alveolar, palato-alveolar, retroflex or glottal voiceless fricative; an alveolar, bilabial nasal or nasalized labio-dental fricative; a mid-open, further open, or slightly centralized front vowel; a VC syllable or a syllabic C.

3.22.5 Finally, under the heading of *unanalyzed,* we give any ad hoc analyses which occur to us of the data left at the foot of the transcriptional page, or which turned out to be unanalysable in the course of profiling. For example, the item *lemon* ['wəʊflə] was given a numbered line, in one sample, as the analyst's first impression was that this was capable of a straightforward analysis. Only when he tried to assign it to its places on the profile chart did he realize that the item contained complications—at which point he transferred the whole item to the unanalysed section on the final supplementary page, returning to it later when all such complex items had been identified. Whether these items yield any interesting findings cannot be predicted; what is important is that one should not waste time attempting to handle them in conventional profile terms. As always in profile work, one should cope with the clear cases first, referring to the unclear cases only if the initial analysis does not provide sufficient grounds for a principled intervention.

3.23* In view of the breadth of information which the supplementary pages can provide, it is perhaps worth emphasizing the point made earlier in this chapter (3.17) that one should be selective and flexible in approaching the task of quantification, for routine clinical purposes. If it is possible to see the nature of P's phonological problem clearly in the configurations of the profile chart, then it may not be necessary to quantify anything (except insofar as one may want to make one's reasoning explicit, for others to see). But when a phonological pattern is unclear, and it is not at all obvious what to do next, then a more detailed analysis of a particular section of the chart may be extremely helpful. As so often, time spent in the preliminary stages of therapy may save time in the long run; but for this to be true, profile procedures must be used intelligently, not mechanically.

We can see this principle in operation if we follow through a small section of the profile chart, from the stage of assessment to that of remedial intervention. The initial plosive system of one P was as follows:

p —	ᴜᴴᴛ ‖		fɪ pᶠ ‖‖	b —	ᴜᴴ‖		m ‖ bβ ‖
	‖		ɸ ᵘ h ‖‖				
t —	ᴜᴴ ‖		κ‖‖ d‖‖ n‖ w ‖	d —	ᴜᴴᴛ ᴜᴴᴛ		t ᴜᴴᴛ d ‖‖ dʒ ‖
	‖		h ‖		‖		
k —			t ᴜᴴᴛ f ‖ 2 ‖	g —	ᴜᴴᴛ ‖‖		b ‖ g ‖‖
			2 ‖‖ h ‖				

It is evident that there is considerable instability in the initial plosive system: there are no omissions, but over half of the phones are errors, as could be shown on the manner target matrix:

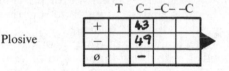

Plosive

	T	C–	–C–	–C
+		43		
–		49		
ø		–		

Let us assume that a decision has already been made (but see further below) to work on initial plosives. T might decide to do some auditory discrimination work in this area, for example. The question is: which pair of phonemes will provide the most fruitful starting-point, and which thereafter? There are 30 possible contrasts to choose from at the outset (/p/ v. /t/, /p/ v. /k/, /p/ v. /b/ etc.); 29 to follow up with; 28 to follow that . . . The first three remedial steps have to be chosen from a total of nearly 25,000 possible discrimination sequences for place of articulation and voicing contrasts. The odds against T picking the best remedial path intuitively are enormous! But by spending a little time going through the data systematically, it is possible to reduce these odds dramatically, and to come up with a handful of promising lines of action.

Given the absence of any correct realizations of initial /k-/, and the frequency with which this phoneme is used in English, an early focus on /k-/ would seem desirable. P can articulate the sound, as is evident from its use elsewhere in the system. But with which other sound should it be contrasted, as a first step in remediation? The chart shows there to be a particular source of confusion between /k-/ and /t-/. It looks as though P 'thinks' of [k] as an allophone of /t-/—in which case he would have no motivation for initiating a contrastive use. Perhaps a good first step would be to work on the auditory discrimination of /t-/ v. /k-/?

There are grounds for doubt about this decision. Scrutiny of the /t-/–/d-/ contrast shows that the feature of voicing is not well established. The facts can be summarized in the voicing matrix:

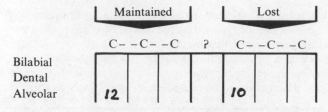

Because of the overlap between /t-/ and /d-/, there is a real danger that, if /k-/ is contrasted with /t-/, P will be uncertain about whether the contrast is being drawn with /t-/ or /d-/. The [t] phone has a high functional load in this system, as reference to the relevant section of the supplementary pages indicates:

Functional
load   [t] ◄── t-, k-, d-

P might go so far as to 'conclude' that, if /k-/ v. /t-/ and /k-/ v. /d-/ are 'the same', therefore the contrast between /t-/ and /d-/ cannot be as important as he might previously have thought it to be. It is conceivable that this might lead to a less efficient control over the voicing feature, and that this might feed back into other positions—perhaps with [k] coming to be used as a realization of /g-/. For this analyst, at any rate, the risk is too great.

As an alternative, what about introducing /k-/ v. /g-/, as an initial remedial step? It is a standard technique, to introduce voiced/voiceless minimal pairs, but there are grounds for doubting the wisdom of such a move in this case. Such a remedial strategy presupposes that P's voicing contrast is fairly well established, and this is not the case, as we have seen. Most of the substitution phones under /g-/ involve voicing problems, which account for the *Lost* total on the voicing matrix:

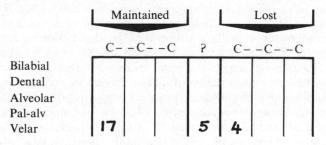

There is also some uncertain voicing under /k-/ (through the use of the glottal stop). It would seem reasonable to work on stabilizing the voiced/voiceless opposition here, if one could rely on the other categories of place and manner of articulation; but there are grounds for distrusting the stability of both of these. The place matrix shows considerable variability, largely associated with /k-/. (The manner substitutions seem less serious at this point—though reference to plosive substitutions elsewhere in the data would complicate the picture.)

−Vel 1 - - 1 - - 5 - - - - - 4 - - 7 - - - - -

With two areas of instability between /k-/ and /g-/, accordingly, this would seem to be a particularly difficult contrast to teach, in the first instance.

A third line of action is more promising: /k-/ v. /p-/. The contrast between /p-/ and /b-/ is well established, with no sign of any voicing confusion:

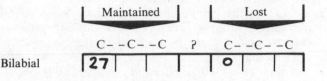

It might therefore be possible to establish a parallelism: /b/ v. /g/ and /p/ v. /k/—which would be a solid foundation for a final step, /k/ vs. /g/. But two possible worries need to be eliminated: (a) both /p/ and /k/ are substituted by [h] in unstressed syllables—which suggests that remedial work should concentrate on stressed contrasts only; (b) there is one /b/–/g/ substitution. Reference to the transcriptional page showed that this was the result of Consonant harmony, the /g/ having fallen under the influence of a preceding /b/, in the phrase *big garden* ['bɪ 'bɑːdə]. T would therefore have to keep an eye on the possibility of perseveration in this direction in the sequences presented to P, and use alternative contexts as required.

Once some motivation for a specific remedial goal has been achieved, the process of teaching may begin, with reference to the usual constraints (of materials, presentation, etc.). At this point, linguistic analysis gives way to therapeutic skills, and a different range of factors arise.

The above example is typical of the kind of reasoning which must take place if arbitrariness in phonological therapy is to be avoided. All too often, the gap between 'P has a problem with initial plosives' and 'I will work on *X* v. *Y*' is bridged with no reasons given. The above discussion does not exhaust the range of reasons which might be adduced to reinforce a particular line of action. In particular, no reference has been made to perceptual limitations. Also, the example is somewhat artificial, in that the decision had already been made to work on initial plosives—but that decision would, in its turn, have had to be scrutinized using similar criteria (why initial plosives, as opposed to other plosives? why plosives, as opposed to other consonant categories? why consonants, as opposed to vowels? and so on). As an illustration of the whole process of reasoning *ab initio*, we therefore conclude this chapter with a case study, of a 4½-year-old language-delayed child (LARSP Stages II–III) with severe phonological problems. A 30-minute sample of his conversation during free play and picture description produced the transcription given below. Quite a wide vocabulary range was produced, but several items are repeated: 115 word types are used on 274 occasions, with 141 repeated forms. There were also very few (17) variant forms, suggestive of a stable and unvarying phonology—*lacking* the variability which one would hope to see in a developing phonology at this stage. Of the intelligible targets, there were few analytical problems (5), but about one-sixth of his speech was not intelligible (52 items). Given his overall intelligibility, in the routine clinical situation we proceeded directly to a target analysis (cf. 3.19); but for present purposes, totals have also been entered into the inventory section of the supplementary pages. This indicates some important biases, especially: a very low C:V ratio (1.14), pointing to a strong open syllable preference; a heavy use of plosives, and a light use of fricatives; a heavy use of alveolar and glottal places of articulation (especially the former); a wide range of vowel types; and very few clusters (also displaying the plosive/alveolar bias).

It is evident from the profile chart that P has rather different consonant systems operating in initial and final position. Initially, plosives are generally correct, whereas finally there is a strong tendency towards omission and glottalization; medially, plosives function sometimes as initial consonants, sometimes as final ones. There is nothing systematic that can be said about affricates, on this evidence: the 5 initial instances are all from a single lexical item (62). Apart from [h-], which is dropped, errors in initial fricatives are in the direction of plosives or affricates; the status of [f-] is ambiguous, as it appears correctly in a limited lexical range (cf. 68). Fricatives are generally absent in final position; medially, they seem to be following the pattern of initial fricatives, being replaced by plosives. Nasals are generally correct in initial position, but there is some omission and overlap in final position. Apart from [j-], initial approximants are poor, generally being replaced by glottal stops or being omitted; final [-l], while somewhat over-articulated, is generally correct. The totals in the target analysis (phones) produce a precise overall statement: in initial position, 69 per cent of consonant phones are correct, with 23 per cent incorrect and 8 per cent omissions; in medial position, the situation is the reverse, with 21 per cent correct, 77 per cent incorrect and 2 per cent omissions; and in final position, there is a different pattern of error again, with 32.5 per cent correct, 32.5 per cent incorrect and 35 per cent omissions. The two main foci of error substitution show up very clearly in the error analysis realizations: a major tendency for alveolar substitutions or glottalization (in the place analysis), and for plosive or affricate substitutions (in the manner analysis). (The problems with final [-l] are not the same kind, and may well contain an element of transcriptional error, in view of the problems involved in hearing 'dark *l*' after certain vowels.) It should be noted, from the feature analysis of voicing, that the voiced/voiceless contrast seems not to be a problem, for this P: in the vast majority of cases, the contrast is being maintained.

P's consonant difficulties should also not obscure the fact that there are several vowel problems. Discounting the substitutions for [əʊ] and [ɛə], which are probably dialectal (see Accent Conventions), we are left with a total of 16 per cent errors in vowel use. The profile shows clearly that these errors are almost entirely located in the front part of the vowel area, and tend to affect adjacent dimensions—for instance, close vowels tend to be substituted by other close vowels; front vowels tend to be substituted by front or central vowels (hardly ever by back); and so on. But the more serious problem is a matter of vowel length. It is the short vowels which are mainly affected, as can be seen from the length matrix in the vowel column—of 38 short vowel errors, 33 involve a lengthening. One should also note, from the diphthongization matrix, that there are 14 cases of monophthongization in the sample. The significance of these points is not solely in relation to vowel articulation: length of vowel is an important aspect of the identification of final consonants in English—final 'voiced' consonants are preceded by longer vowels than final 'voiceless' ones. In view of P's weakness in final position, the remedial work in this area would need to bear this vowel-consonant interaction in mind. (Presumably, for example, consonant discrimination would be aided, to begin with, if maximally contrasting vowels were used, e.g. *sit* v. *sad*, as opposed to *sit* v. *Sid*.) Nor should the issue be seen in isolation from P's rhythmic skills. These were rudimentary: he was unable to copy correctly sequences of 3 claps to different rhythms, for example. In the present sample, there were only a few instances of wrong stress patterns on words, but the general impression of P's speech was of an erratic rhythm, and this would complicate any work on vowel length in connected speech. Indeed, the logic of the argument 'consonant confusion → vowel length confusion → erratic rhythmic skills' would suggest that systematic work on rhythm should be an early remedial aim, and could have pervasive results.

The process analysis shows that P's consonant problems are not just matters of simple substitution. There are several cases where perseveration and other sequencing difficulties emerge. There are some ambiguous cases, but in most of the relevant examples, the direction of the assimilation is strongly progressive: an initial consonant influences a medial or final one. It should be noted that, in every case, the focus of the influence is alveolar—usually [t] or [d]. There is no known physiological reason for P's bias towards these sounds, but they are a major cause of the ambiguity of P's speech, as is evident from the functional load line on the final page of the chart, where [t] and [d] each expound 12 target phones. It is plain that a massive systematization of P's sound system would take place if progress could be made in restricting P's alveolar plosive bias. This, along with the major weakness in initial approximants (a severe aspect of P's overall delay), seem to be the most plausible topics for early remediation.

Phonological Profile (PROPH)

Name James S.
Age 4;6   Sample date 24.2.81

Duration 30 mins.
Type Free play & picture description

Accent conventions   modified RP (Berks.) əʊ → oʊ   ɛə → ɛː

Gloss	Transcriptions		Gloss	Transcriptions
it	ɪʔ ‖‖ ɪh ǀ ɪk ǀ		in	ɪn ‖‖ ɪː ǀ
on	ɒn ‖⫢‖		the	ðə ‖⫢
there	ðɛː ‖⫢ dɛː ‖		no	'noʊ ‖⫢ ‖⫢ ‖⫢ ‖ 'ʔoʊ ǀ
I	'aɪ ‖⫢			
a	ə ‖‖			
he	i ‖‖			
yeah	ɛː ǀ jɛh ‖⫢			

Gloss	Transcriptions		Gloss	Transcriptions		Gloss	Transcriptions
1 tortoise	'tɔːtɪ		41 pink	'pʰɪŋ		81 straw	'tʃaː
2 slowly	'toʊdeɪ		42 go	'goʊ ‖‖		82 naughty	'ʔɔːʔiː
3 wake	'wɪʔ		43 where	'wɛː		83 turkey	'tɜːtiː ‖‖
4 up	'ʌh		44 too	'tuː		84 sheep	'tsɪː ǀ tʰɪ ǀ
5 daisy	'deɪdiː		45 none	'nʌn		85 stick	'dɪ
6 white	'aɪ ‖		46 look	'lɒʔ		86 camera	'kænkaː
7 grey	'ʔeɪ ‖		47 brown	'baʊ		87 lamb	'æn
8 bandy	'bændiː ‖		48 postman	'poʊmən		88 milkman	'mɪlmən
9 eat	'iːt ‖ iː² ǀ		49 garage	'dædɪ		89 post	'poʊʔ
10 mice	'maɪ		50 nothing	'nʌdɪŋ		90 letter	'ʔetaː
11 fish	'ʧi		51 shepherd	'ʧeptʰə		91 digging	'dɪdˀɪŋ
12 dog	'dɒ ‖ 'dɒʔ ǀ		52 car	'kaː		92 red	'ʔeɪ ʔ
13 bone	'boʊ ‖		53 fall	'tɔː(ꞁ)		93 window	'ʔɪndoʊ
14 cat	'kæh		54 lamp-post	'ʔæmpoʊh		94 teacake	'tiːkeɪ
15 sooty	'tuː 'ʔiː		55 bedroom	'bedɹuː		95 goldfish	'goʊd 'ʧɪ
16 blue	'bˡuː ‖		56 inside	'ɪntaɪ		96 little	'ʔɪˀl ‖‖ 'ʔɪːʔəl ǀ
17 orange	'ɒwɪn⃝		57 can	'kæn		97 pig	'pɪ ‖⫢
18 ribbons	ɪ'dɪnz		58 outside	'æntaɪ		98 cow	'kaʊ ‖⫢
19 more	'mɔː ‖		59 top	'tɒ		99 horsie	'ɔːtiː ‖‖ 'ɔːʔiː ‖
20 green	'giː		60 roof	'ʔʊts 'ʔuːh		100 farm	'paːm
21 oh	'oʊ		61 house	'aʊts 'ʔaʊ			
22 egg	'eg		62 chicken	'ʧɪʧɪn ‖‖			Problems
23 bowl	'boʊ		63 quack	'kæ ‖		cabbage	'kædʒɪ
24 putting	'pʊtɪŋ 'pʊʔɪn		64 baby	'beɪbiː		Catford	'kæbtʃuː
25 table	'teːtəl		65 one	'ʌn		duck(s)?	'dʌ ‖
26 cake	'keɪ		66 two	'tuː ‖		farmer	'paːmæn
27 tea	'tiː		67 three	'fʷiː		dunno	noʊ ‖⫢ ǀ
28 butter	'bʌtaː		68 four	'fɔː ‖			noʊ ǀ
29 jam	'jæŋ 'dʒæʔ		69 they	ðeɪ ǀ			dn̩'noʊ ‖
30 mine	'maɪn		70 friends	'ten			
31 sugar	'tˢuːtaː		71 hiding	'aɪdɪ ǀ			
32 milk	'mɪl		72 found	'taʊn ǀ			
33 fork	'fɔː		73 down	'daʊn ǀ 'ʔaʊn ǀ			
34 knife	'naɪ		74 stay	'deɪ			
35 girl	'ʔɜː(ꞁ)		75 field	'fiːəl			
36 boy	'bɔɪ		76 home	'ʔoʊm			
37 daddy	'dædiː ‖		77 eating	'iːtɪŋ			
38 mummy	'mʌmiː		78 some	'tʌn			
39 bigger	'bɪgʌ		79 food	'tuː			
40 big	'bɪ 'bɪʔ		80 bread	'bed			

Total word types	115		TTR	·42
Total word tokens	274		Total problems	5
Repeated forms	141		Total unintelligible	52
Variant forms	17		Analysed:unanalysed	·79

C –

p–	10	pʰ 1 / p̃ 1		b–	14		
t–	13			d–	11	2 2	
k–	11 / 1			g–	6	ᵈ 1	
tʃ–	5			dʒ–	1	j 1	
f–	5	ɟ̇2 t4 pⁱ		v–			
θ–				ð–	2 / 12	d 3	
s–		t 2 / t 2		z–			
ʃ–		ɟ̇1 tʃ 3 tʃ 1					
h–	11	2 2					
				m–	8 / 2		
				n–	21	2 3	
w–	2	4	21	r–		1	2 3 / 1
j–	6	1		l–	1	1	2 9 / d 1

V

I	22 / 31	ɪː 2 / ɪ: 2 / ɪ: 22 / ɪː 11 əɪ 1		ʊ	1	uː 2 / ʊ 1 ɒ 1
e	6	eɪ 1		ʌ	7		
æ	18 / 2			ɒ	6 / 8		
ə	7	ɪ 2 ɑ 3 / ʌ 1 ʌ 1					
i:	10	ɪ 1 / ɪ: 2		ɜ:	5		
ɑ:	2			u:	9 / 1	ʊ 1	
				ɔ:	18	aɪ 1	
eɪ	9	ɪ 1 / ɛ: 1		ɔɪ	1		
aɪ	9 / 2			eə			
əʊ		ɒʊ 32 / ɒʊ 1		ɔɪə			
əʊə				aɪə			
aʊə				aʊ	15	æ 1	
ɪə	1			ɛə			
						ɛ: 1 / ɛ: 3 / ɛ: 10 eh 5	

| ə | 5 | I/i: | 5 | ʊ/u: | | ɑ:/aʊə | | æ/ɜ: | |
| əʊ | 1 | eɪ | | aɪ | 6 | ɪə | | ɛə | |

CC –

p	l–			b	l–	bˡ 3		θ	r–	ⓔʷ 1	
	r–				r–	b 2			j–		
	j–				w–				w		
t	r–			d	r–			ʃ	l–		
	j–				j–				r–	t 1	
	w–				w–				j–		
k	l–			g	l–			m	j–		
	r–				r–	23 91		n			
	j–				j–			l			
	w–	k 3			w–			h			
								v			
s	p–			s	l–	t 1		s	w–		
	t–	d 2			m–				j–		
	k–				n–			ʃ	r–		

Stress

ˌ		◡/ 1	
	60	// 2	
ˈ ˌ			
ˌ ˌ			
3+			

CCC –

s	p	l–			s	t	r–	tʃ 1		s	k	l–		
		r–					j–					r–		
		j–										j–		
												w–		

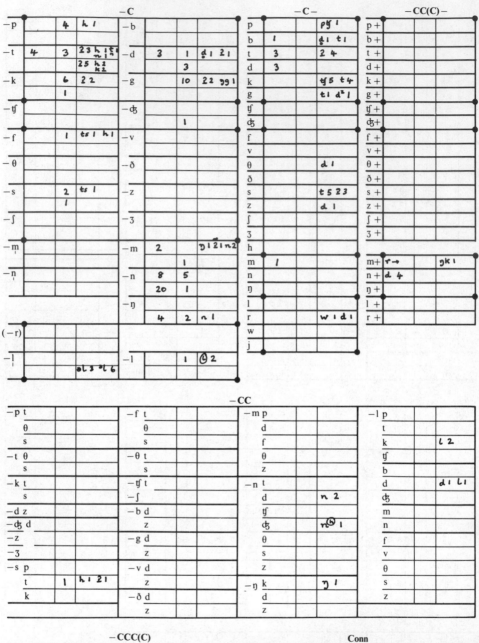

Inventory of Phones   Consonants

Place

	Bil	L-d	Den	Alv	P-al	Ret	Pal-a	Pal	Vel	Uvu	Pha	Glo	Oth
C	46	5	15	148	1	-	15	7	31	-	-	57	-
CC	4	1	-	7	-	-	-	-	2	-	-	-	-
CC	1	-	-	10	-	-	1	-	2	-	-	-	-
Tot	51	6	15	165	1	-	16	7	35	-	-	57	-

		Total C-	176
		Total -C-	37
		Total -C	87

Manner

	Plo	Aff	Fric	Nas	App	Other Pul	Other Non-pul
C	173	19	31	76	26	-	-
CC	6	-	1	7	-	-	-
CC	6	1	3	-	4	-	-
Tot	185	20	35	83	30	-	-

Total C	353
Total V	310
C:V	1·14

Target Analysis (Phones)   Error Analysis Realizations

Place

	T	C-	-C-	-C		Bil	Den	Alv	P-a	Vel	Glo	Tot
Bilabial +	40	36	2	2								
Bilabial −	11	3	3	5	−Bil	2 ... 2 2 ... 1 1 ... 2 ... 1						
Bilabial ø	9	4	0	5								
(Labio-)Dental +	19	19	0	0								
(Labio-)Dental −	13	10	1	2	−Den	1 ... 7 1 ... 2 ... 1 ... 1						
(Labio-)Dental ø	1	0	0	1								
Alveolar +	88	47	6	35								
Alveolar −	66	22	15	29	−Alv	− 1 ... 5 7 15 ... 2 17 7 12 ...						
Alveolar ø	20	2	1	17								
Palato-alveolar +	12	12	0	0								
Palato-alveolar −	6	6	0	0	−P-a	... 4 ... 2 ...						
Palato-alveolar ø	4	1	0	3								
Velar +	23	18	0	5								
Velar −	18	1	11	6	Vel	... 1 6 1 ... 5 ... 1 ... 4 ...						
Velar ø	19	0	0	19								
Glottal +	0	0	0									
Glottal −	2	2	0		−Glo	... 2 ...						
Glottal ø	11	11	0									
Total +	182	132	8	42								
Total −	116	44	30	42	−Tot	3 1 0 0 0 0 17 16 18 4 5 0 0 0 4 20 7 19 0 1 1						
Total ø	64	18	1	45								

Manner

	T	C-	C-	C		Plo	Aff	Fric	Nas	App	Other
Plosive +	81	66	7	8							
Plosive −	46	5	18	23	−Plo	5 11 17 ... 6 ... 4 ... 1 ... 1 1					
Plosive ø	29	0	1	28							
Affricate +	6	6	0	0							
Affricate −	1	1	0	0	−Aff	... 1 ...					
Affricate ø	1	0	0	1							
Fricative +	19	19	0	0							
Fricative −	34	21	10	3	−Fric	15 10 ... 6 ... 2 ... 1 ...					
Fricative ø	17	11	0	6							
Nasal +	66	31	1	34							
Nasal −	8	3	0	5	−Nas	3 ... 5 ...					
Nasal ø	9	0	0	9							
Approximant +	10	10	0	0							
Approximant −	27	14	2	11	−App	14 1 ... 1 11 ...					
Approximant ø	8	7	0	1							
Total +	182	132	8	42							
Total −	116	44	30	42	−Tot	37 22 17 6 6 2 0 0 5 0 0 6 1 1 11 0 1 1					
Total ø	64	18	1	45							

Vowels

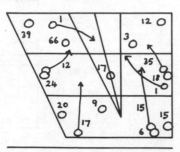

Error Analysis Realizations

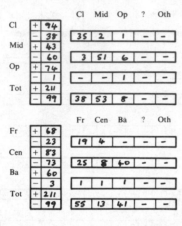

		Cl	Mid	Op	?	Oth
Cl	+ 94					
	− 38	35	2	1	−	−
Mid	+ 43					
	− 60	3	51	6	−	−
Op	+ 74					
	− 1	−	−	1	−	−
Tot	+ 211					
	− 99	38	53	8	−	−

		Fr	Cen	Ba	?	Oth
Fr	+ 68					
	− 23	19	4	−	−	−
Cen	+ 83					
	− 73	25	8	40	−	−
Ba	+ 60					
	− 3	1	1	1	−	−
Tot	+ 211					
	− 99	55	13	41	−	−

	V	VV(V)	Other
V	43	2	0
VV(V)	14	34	6

	Oral	Nasal	?
Oral	98	1	0

	V́	Ṽ	?
V́	0	1	0
Ṽ	3	0	0

	Roun	Unr	?
Roun	5	1	0
Unr	0	39	0

	V	V:	?
V	5	33	0
V:	2	3	0

Inventory of Clusters

	I	M	F
CC	4	6	4
CCC(C)	−	−	−

Place	Bil	Den	Alv	Pal-a	Vel	Oth	Tot
Bilabial	−	−	3	1	−	−	−
Dental	1	−	−	−	−	−	−
Alveolar	−	−	7	−	−	−	−
Pal-alv	−	−	−	−	−	−	−
Velar	−	−	−	−	2	−	−
Other	−	−	−	−	−	−	−
Total	1	0	10	1	2	0	0

Manner	Plo	Aff	Fric	Nas	App	Oth	Tot
Plosive	−	1	2	−	3	−	−
Affricate	−	−	−	−	−	−	−
Fricative	−	−	−	−	1	−	−
Nasal	6	−	1	−	−	−	−
Approx	−	−	−	−	−	−	−
Other	−	−	−	−	−	−	−
Total	6	1	3	0	4	0	0

Target Analysis (Clusters)

	I	M	F
CC(CC)	4	5	2
C > CC	0	1	3
CC > +V	0	0	0
$C_1C_2 > C_1$	6	0	6
$C_1C_2 > C_2$	0	0	1
$C_1C_2 > C_3$	7	0	2

	I	M	F
CC > ø	0	1	0
CCC > C_4	1	0	0

Place	Bil +	Bil −	Den +	Den −	Alv +	Alv −	Pal-a +	Pal-a −	Vel +	Vel −	Oth −	Total +	Total −
Bilabial	−	−	−	−	3	1	−	−	+	−	−	3	1
Dental	−	−	−	−	−	1	−	−			−	−	1
Alveolar	−	−	−	−	5	−	−	/	−	−	−	5	1
Pal-alv					−	/					−	−	−
Velar	−	−			−	−	−	−	−	−	−	−	−
Glottal					−	−					−	−	−
Total	−	−	−	−	8	2	−	/	−	−			

Manner	Plo +	Plo −	Aff +	Aff −	Fric +	Fric −	Nas +	Nas −	App +	App −	Oth −	Total +	Total −
Plosive	−	−			−	−			3	−	−	3	−
Affricate	−	−									−	−	/
Fricative	−	−			−	−	−	−	−	/	−	−	/
Nasal	4	−	−	/	1	−	1	−	−	/	−	5	2
Approx	−	−	−	−	−	−	−	−	−	−	−	−	−
Total	4	−	−	/	1	−	−	−	3	2	−		

Feature Analysis (Phones)

Voicing

Place	Maintained				Lost			Maintained	Lost	Maintained	Lost
	C–	–C–	–C	?	C–	–C–	–C	C– –C– –C	C– –C– –C	C– –C– –C	C– –C– –C
Bilabial	38	3	6	2	–	2	–				
Dental	29	–	2	–	–	1	–				
Alveolar	52	14	53	33	–	–	2				
Pal-alv	18	–	–	–	–	–	–				
Velar	19	10	7	4	–	1	–				
Glottal	–	–	–	2	–	–	–				
Total	156	27	68	41	–	4	2				

Manner

	C–	–C–	–C	?	C–	–C–	–C				
Plosive	69	18	16	19	–	3	2				
Affricate	7	–	–	–	–	–	–				
Fricative	38	6	3	5	–	1	–				
Nasal	31	1	38	4	–	–	–				
Approximant	11	2	11	13	–	–	–				
Total	156	27	68	41	–	4	2				

Feature Analysis (Clusters)

Voicing

	Maintained	Lost	Other
CC–	4	–	–
–CC–	4	1	–
–CC	1	1	–
Total	9	2	–

Process Analysis

Syllable Structure

S Deletion

S Addition

C Deletion

C Addition   ʔæntaʃ (58)

Other   Reversals (11, 95 [ʧɪʃ])
        ? cabbage, Catford

Assimilations

C Harmony
(2, 5, 25, 31, 49, 51, 54, 62,
83, 91   ? 15, 18, 50, 82)

V Harmony
(18, 28)

Other

Substitutions

?   86

Functional load
[t] → t–, f–, s–, ʃ–, sl–, fr–, –t, –b–, –t–, –k–, –g–, –s–
[d] → d–, g–, ð–, l–, st–, –d, –ld, –b–, –g–, –θ–, –z–, –r–
[ʒ] → d–, n–, w–, r–, l–, gr–, –t, –d, –k, –g, –m, –st, –t–, –s–

Variants   t/ʒ   ʒ/∅   ð/d

Contrasts 100% +
p–/t–/k–/ɥ–   k–/g–   b–/d–   ?p–/b–   ?–t–/–d–
m–/n–   ɥ–/dʒ–   b–/g–   ?t–/d–

100% –
–t/–d   –k/–g   –p/–t   –r–/–w–   ?w–/r–/l–   ?–m/–n/–ŋ   –t–/–k–/–g–/–s–

Indeterminacy
C   l

V

Syll

Unanalysed   See p. 1.

4 PROP

4.1* The nonsegmental phonological profile known as PROP ('*Pro*sody *Pro*file') is a single-page chart, on which can be placed information about the main prosodic patterns encountered in a sample of clinical data. The term 'prosody' here refers to the *linguistic* use of pitch, loudness, speed of speech, pause, and rhythm—in other words, to the way in which these variables can alter the meaning of what we say. PROP is not intended for the description of *phonetic* abnormalities in the use of these variables, as will be found under the heading of 'voice disorders' (in relation to the term *dysprosody,* for example). PROP is an aspect of *phonological* analysis, complementing the analysis of the segmental aspects of pronunciation carried out in Chapter 3.

4.2 While in principle any of the prosodic variables of speech could be disturbed, and contribute to P's communication problems, in practice it is *pitch* which causes most linguistic difficulties, and the bulk of the profile chart is therefore given over to an analysis of this variable. The linguistic use of pitch is usually referred to as *intonation,* and indeed it is intonation with which we are most regularly concerned, in clinical settings. But other prosodic factors need to be related to intonation, if a full understanding of P's difficulties is to emerge—and in any case, we need to be able to note the occurrence of other categories of prosodic problem, if the principle of profile comprehensiveness is to be maintained (cf. 1.9). There is therefore space on the chart for a reference to other things than intonation (see further, 4.8).

4.3* The intonational theory which the chart reflects recognizes 3 main distinctions in the way pitch patterns are used in a language: the organization of connected speech into *tone units;* the use of specific *tones* within these units; and the phenomenon of *tonicity,* within these units. Distinct patterns of disorder are associated with each of these notions, but first their normal use in relation to English needs to be explained.

4.3.1 The primary organization of speech is into *tone units* (sometimes called *tone groups*). A tone unit is a finite set of pitch movements, grouped into a distinctive contour and uttered with a distinctive rhythm. Tone units are often bounded by pauses, and these boundaries generally coincide with points of grammatical junction. A tone-unit boundary is marked with a slant line, in this system of transcription, as follows:

> *if you see him/ ask him to call/*
> *I'd like to buy some eggs/ a pint of milk/ and some butter/*
> *the dog bit the cat/ and the cat bit the dog/*

Prosody Profile (PROP)

Name	Duration
Age	Sample date	Type

Tone Unit (0; 9 +)   Total   Average words

Structures

Incomplete	Indeterminate	Stereotyped	Imitation
Clause		**Functions**	
Phrase			
Word			
Other Cl +			
Cl −			

Tone (0; 9 +)

Data   Variants

Deviant

Summary: Other   N   W   ↓   ?↑   ↑   ‖   ∅

		Other	N	W	↓	?↑	↑	‖	∅
0; 9 +	−								
	`								
1; 0 +	´								
1; 3 +	^								
	ˇ								
1; 6 +	C								
	?								

Tonicity (1; 6 +)

	Indeterminate	Stereotyped	Imitation

	Non Final		Final	
	✓	×	✓	×
Simple				
Lexical				
Grammatical				
Complex	NF + NF		NF + F	

Other

Tone unit pitch	Prosodic features (TU +)
Tone unit other	Paraling features

There are several constraints governing the distribution of tone units in most conversational speech; but in certain circumstances, these constraints may be ignored. In very fast speech, for example, tone units run together and lose their clear relationship to grammar. And in highly emotional speech, each word may be given a separate tone unit, e.g.

I/ said/ do/ it/ now/ .

Several types of linguistic disability can be characterized by disturbances in the normal production or comprehension of the tone unit structure of speech.

4.3.2 One of the main characteristics of a tone unit is that its pitch contour achieves a peak of prominence, through the use of one of a small number of *tones*. While every syllable in a tone unit must be uttered on some tone (i.e. given a specific pitch level or movement), one syllable's tone always stands out more than the others, and this is referred to as the *nuclear tone* (the syllable carrying it being known as the *tonic* syllable). The normal place for the tonic syllable is towards the end of the tone unit (see futher, 4.7.1), but it may be brought forward onto almost any other word, if grammatical or semantic factors allow it. Tonic placement, or *tonicity,* changes the emphasis within a tone unit, and usually introduces a fresh contrast in meaning, as in the following examples:

John saw Mary in *town/*
John saw *Mary* in town/ (as opposed to someone else)
John saw Mary in town/ (as opposed to someone else)
John *saw* Mary in town/ (but he didn't talk to her)

4.3.3* Under the heading of *tone* is analysed the direction and range of pitch carried by the tonic syllable. Three types of nuclear tone are recognized in the present approach: *simple, complex* and *compound.* Simple tones are the three possibilities of unidirectional pitch movement—falling tones (ˋ), rising tones (ˊ) and level tones (ˉ). Complex tones are all nuclei where there is a change in direction of the pitch movement within a syllable, the main categories of English being the falling-rising (ˇ) and rising-falling (ˆ) tones. Compound tones are combinations of certain of the above tones used on different syllables within a tone unit, but acting as if they were a *single* tone, e.g. a combination of a falling tone with a rising tone produces a 'fall-plus-rise'. Examples of these tones are given below (with just one possible interpretation of the attitudinal meaning conveyed by the tone). The typographical convention is to place the accent mark over the vowel of the stressed syllable in a word.

John's còming/	(neutral; matter-of-fact)
John's cóming/	(questioning, surprised, if the tone has a high end-point)
John's cōming/	(routine, bored)
John's cǒming/	(warning, caution)
John's côming/	(definite, impressed)
Jòhn's cóming/	(extra emphasis on *John*)
Jóhn's còming/	(extra emphasis on *John*)

The average percentage frequency of occurrence of these tones in adult conversational English is as follows:

` 51.2;  ´ 20.8;  ˇ 8.5;  ` + ´ 7.7; ^ 5.2; ‾ 4.9; ´ + ` 1.7

Nuclear tones signal both attitudinal and grammatical information. Examples of the former are given above; examples of the latter would include the distinction between utterance end v. utterance continuation, signalled by tones which end in a falling direction v. tones which end in a rising direction, e.g.

  'would you like cóffee/ or tèa/
  'would you like cóffee/ or téa/

In the first case, two alternatives are being offered, and no more; whereas in the second case, there are further, unmentioned possibilities.

4.3.4 Other prosodic distinctions may need to be referred to upon occasion, and it is helpful to have available a detailed system of transcription to provide the necessary support. In particular, use is often made of the following:

'	a stressed syllable, where the prominence is due to extra loudness, and not to a step-up or step-down in pitch;
''	a stronger degree of stress;
↑	a noticeable step-up in pitch, compared with the pitch level of the preceding syllable;
↓	a noticeable step-down in pitch, compared with the pitch level of the preceding syllable;
' '	are used to include a stretch of utterance characterized by some prosodic feature, such as extra height, slow speed, marked rhythm; the explanation of the inverted commas is given in the margin of the transcription;
–	a pause equivalent to a beat of the speaker's normal conversational rhythm; longer pauses are marked accordingly, viz. – –, – – –;
.	a brief pause, shorter than a speaker's rhythm unit.

4.4* While very little empirical research into the acquisition of prosodic features has been carried out, it is nonetheless possible to establish some general developmental principles, and these are reflected in the vertical organization of the chart. The earliest sign of intonational organization in the vocalization of an infant is the emergence of a basic rhythm/pitch unit, which is sometimes to be heard from about 6 months, but which is usually well in evidence by 9 months. The chunking of the child's vocalization into these units is often quite striking, and is usually interpreted by listening adults as attempts by the child to 'say something'. It is important to note that the prosodic shape which these chunks of vocalization manifest is a definable and stable phenomenon long before the child's utterance takes on a stable *segmental* phonological form. Certainly by 12 months, in most children, tone units, in the sense of 4.3, are well established as a means of organizing speech—whether the speech be 'one word sentences' or an unintelligible 'jargon'. The first section of the profile chart is therefore given over to the development of tone units, the classification of which is explained below (4.5).

4.4.1 Specific tonal patterns are of course part of the identity of tone units, and the language-specific use of a tone will be noticed at the same time as the primitive tone units referred to above. But it takes a much longer period of time before the set of tonal contrasts comes to be established—the nuclear tones of mature speech. The main types of nuclear tone seem to emerge between 9 months and 18 months, in English, and the specific order of emergence suggested by the empirical studies of recent years is given in the middle section of the chart. The ordering is tentative, but plausible (see further, 4.6.2).

4.4.2 As tonicity involves a contrast between words in a single tone unit, it is a notion which cannot be relevant until the development of multi-word sentences. Two-word sentences emerge at or around 18 months, and some kind of contrastive emphasis seems to be there from the outset. Tonicity variations are classified in the lower third of the chart; they are discussed further below (4.7).

4.4.3 It is not possible, in the present state of knowledge, to assign any sort of developmental ordering to the other features of tone unit structure, or to other prosodic variables than intonation. These, along with certain other nonsegmental characteristics of speech, are summarized under the heading of *Other* at the bottom of the chart (see further, 4.8). No developmental sequence is given.

4.5* *Tone units*   The most important function of tone units is grammatical— the integration and delimitation of grammatical patterns. The primary focus of attention, therefore, is on the way in which tone units relate to grammatical structure. But there are certain preliminary considerations.

(a) Only *complete* tone units are analysed in terms of grammatical structure. Incomplete tone units are counted separately, and not given any further classification, in the first instance. Examples of incomplete tone units are as follows:

P   he 'said he's ———
P   it's a ———
P   I 'see him ———

From this last example, it should be noted that an utterance may, superficially, look like a complete sentence; but the point is that it does not *sound* like one, from an intonational point of view. The utterance sounds unfinished—perhaps because it suddenly stops short, or because it drawls slowly into silence. There may be several incomplete tone units in a single sequence, as P attempts a sentence several times, e.g.

P   he's ——— I 'think he's ——— he's ——

Each bit of speech in this example sounded like a fresh start at an utterance. Each bit had its own rhythm and pitch, and was clearly surrounded by pauses.

It was therefore counted as three incomplete tone units. This kind of pattern is repeatedly found in the nonfluent P presented in 4.9.

If one were not sure about whether a tone unit were complete or not, the right course of action would be to place the piece of utterance concerned under the next category on the chart.

(b) Indeterminate tone units are those where there are grounds for uncertainty as to whether a complete tone unit has been produced. This commonly happens when people are talking rapidly, and it becomes very difficult to hear to what extent prosody is structuring their utterance at all. Vaguely discernable rhythm units may be present, but that is all. Under such circumstances, all one can do is assign each identifiable chunk of speech to the *indeterminate* category. Similarly, if P is talking and T intervenes, thus talking at the same time as P, and making it difficult to hear how or whether P finished off his utterance, it would be unclear whether a tone unit was complete or not, and the *indeterminate* category should again be used. Certain types of disability are likely to manifest large numbers of indeterminate (and incomplete) tone units—for example, cluttering and stuttering, or some of the slurred speech characteristic of neurological patients. But it must not be forgotten that uncertainty about tone unit status is a perfectly normal phenomenon, if there is a reduction in the phonetic cues, for any reason (e.g. an unclear pitch contour, or abnormal hesitancy). (Conversely, a tone unit may be clearly identifiable, even though its segmental/verbal content is unintelligible.)

(c) Stereotyped prosodic patterns are also encountered—a fixed rhythm and pitch contour for a particular stretch or utterance. Nursery rhymes, limericks and proverbs illustrate everyday examples of stereotyped prosody. In the context of disability, however, any piece of speech may come to be used in this way. For example, one aphasic P would say *very nice thank-you*, not always appropriately, to many T stimuli, but always with the same prosodic pattern. In much the same way as one would, on the LARSP chart, assign this utterance to the Stereotyped box (cf. 2.5.2), here too one does not analyse it further. Each tone unit which seems to have a fixed internal prosodic structure is assigned to this category. It should be noted that it is the *prosodic form* which is stereotyped—there may be some lexical or grammatical variability. For instance, one P would habitually divide some utterances into two tone units—the first with a high rising tone; the second with a low falling tone, e.g.

he ↑ wánts/ – a 'new ↓ càr/
a ↑ mán/ – on a ↓ bìcycle/

This was only done in certain contexts, such as answering questions about a picture. It was almost as if he had learned a special speech style for responding to such questions. In free conversation settings, there was no sign of this 'antithetical' prosody. The tone units were therefore counted as stereotypes.

(d) When P imitates T, it is often unclear whether P understands what is being said, or is in real control over the utterance. This principle applies as much to prosody as to other aspects of language. T may say a phrase in a nice bouncy intonation, and P imitates it. Because such 'echoes' do not necessarily

tell us anything about P's real control of intonation, they are therefore counted separately, under *Imitation* in this section. Obviously, a decision that there has been prosodic imitation will be clear only if the prosodic patterns used fall well outside of what we would normally expect for P. If T used a tone unit which is within P's capabilities, and P repeats it, one would normally give P the 'credit' for the prosody, and analyse it accordingly. Occasionally, there are cases of doubt—in which case, these would be placed under *imitation*, and not given any subsequent analysis.

These are the various kinds of problem one encounters in extracting the tone units from a sample of data. They are left on one side, and not subsequently analysed—unless, that is, the remainder of the data is so unclear that one is forced to look at them again. But this rarely happens.

4.5.1 All remaining utterances are analysed directly in terms of the general type of grammatical structure they contain.

(a) Under *clause* are placed instances of tone units whose grammatical structure is one or other of the clause units as defined in LARSP (cf. 2.8.1). In the following examples, each tone unit is equivalent to a clause:

> 'man gòing/
> 'where 'man góne/
> the 'cat 'bit the dòg/
> 'when he cómes/ 'I'll be òut/
> 'what he did yésterday/ 'doesn't concèrn me/
> 'put the 'book dòwn/ be'fore you 'pick up the pèn/
> 'I'll 'go tomórrow/ and 'you 'go the nèxt day/

It is normal for uncomplicated clauses, such as *the cat is chasing the dog,* to be produced in a single tone unit.

(b) Under *phrase* are placed instances of tone units whose grammatical structure is one or other of the phrase units as defined in LARSP (cf. 2.8.3). In the following examples, each tone unit is equivalent to a phrase:

> the mán/ is kícking/ a bàll/
> a 'big càt/
> a 'cat in a hàt/
> 'mummy and dàddy/
> and a 'big báll/
> sìt down/
> 'all the péople/ lóoked at/ the pìcture/

(c) Under *word* are placed instances of tone units whose grammatical structure is a single word (whatever its morphological complexity). In the following examples, each tone unit is equivalent to a word:

> yès/   lòok/
> sǒrry/   wàlking/
> mùmmy/   ridìculous/
> gôsh/   mán/ ís/ wàlking/
> thé/ mán/ ís/ kícking/ thé/ bàll/

(d) Under *Other* is placed any use of a tone unit where the internal grammatical structure is not neatly equivalent to one or other of the above three types. Two subtypes are recognized. When a tone unit contains a structure *larger* than a single clause, it is marked under Cl+. When it contains a structure *smaller* than a single clause, but not equivalent to a phrase, it is marked under Cl−. Some examples are:

Cl+:   *I knòw he'll be hére/*
       I 'couldn't 'come I 'had a còld/
       'what I 'said was 'what I mèant/
       when I 'left the hòuse the 'man/ shŏuted. . .
       yes I thìnk so/
Cl−:   *'that man ís/ an ìdiot/*
       'man is kìcking a/ bàll to 'me/
       'where áre/ you gòing/

4.5.2* It should be noted that each utterance is analysed into tone units in strict sequence, with no initial decision being made about the grammatical status of the speech. Combinations of the above patterns therefore are to be found. Here are some 'mixed' examples, assigned to their profile category:

thé/ 'man is kícking/ a bàll/
Word   Cl−   Phrase
'when he cómes/ I rĕally/ dón't/ wánt/ to sèe him/
       Clause   Cl−   Word Word   Cl−

Here is a stretch of dialogue, analysed according to its tone-unit structure (both T and P utterances are analysed in this example, for purposes of illustration):

T   'what are you 'going to dò in the 'holidays/ −−−
                     Clause
P   'open my prèsent 'up/ on 'Christmas Dáy/
            Cl−   *Phrase*
T   'open your prèsent/ .
         Clause
      ôh/
      Word
P   'very exci . ex . excìted/ −
            Phrase   *(the nonfluency here did not seem*
                                        to interfere with the rhythmic
T   yòu áre/   *structure of the unit)*
      Clause
P   erm yès/
            Word
      erm − 'at 'Christmas Dáy/
                  Phrase
T   what èlse do you 'do on 'Christmas 'Day/ −−
                     Clause

P   Chrìstmas . 'present and dínner/ – – –
           Phrase
    and . 'play with 'my . Chrìstmas présent/ –
           Clause

T   'what do you 'think you're 'going to gèt/
           Cl+

P   a bìke/
    Phrase

T   do you knòw that you're 'going to 'get a bíke/ – –
           Cl+

P   yès/
    Word

T   ôh/ – –
    Word

     'where will you rìde/ –
     Clause

P   don't knòw/ – –
    Stereo

4.5.3* Some typical distributions in the tone-unit section of the chart are given in the following summaries:

Tone Unit (0; 9+)				Total		Average words	
Structures							
Incomplete	4	Indeterminate	2	Stereotyped	1	Imitation	0
Clause	50			**Functions**			
Phrase	20						
Word	30						
Other Cl+	10						
Cl–	5						

This is a fairly normal distribution: the majority of the speaker's tone units follow the grammar, with bias towards clause integrity; there are only 5 cases where the intonation has broken up the internal structure of the clause; reference to the grammatical analysis would clarify whether the 30 Word units were predictable (e.g. *yès/, nò/*) or abnormal (e.g. *thé/ mán/ ìs/. . .*).

This pattern can be contrasted with the following, taken from a language-delayed child of 3½:

Tone Unit (0; 9+)				Total		Average words	
Structures							
Incomplete	6	Indeterminate	2	Stereotyped	1	Imitation	1
Clause	9			**Functions**			
Phrase	45						
Word	50						
Other Cl+	0						
Cl–	24						

There are few clausal tone units. Reference to the grammatical analysis would show that this is *not* because there are few clauses: his sample contains over 20 clauses, but they are not produced with a coherent prosodic structure. The high total for Word reflects a Stage I bias in LARSP terms—many single-element · sentences. Similarly, the high Phrase total reflects the preponderance of phrases used in the sample—though here too, not all the phrases are given a coherent prosodic structure. The high figure for *Cl−* also reflects the child's uncertain prosody.

A further pattern can be seen in the following, taken from a 'fluent' aphasic man:

Tone Unit (0; 9+)			Total	Average words
Structures				
Incomplete 20	Indeterminate 23	Stereotyped 15	Imitation 0	
Clause 15		**Functions**		
Phrase 12				
Word 5				
Other Cl+ 41				
Cl− 9				

The most noticeable feature here is the high figure under Cl+, with clause sequences often being subsumed under a single tone unit, clause fragments being attached to clauses (e.g. *it's 'dinner time and èating/*) and sequences of social minor sentences (e.g. *well oh yês/*). The incompleteness, indeterminateness and stereotypicality of fluent aphasic speech is well attested, and it manifests itself particularly clearly on a prosodic profile.

4.5.4* Tone-unit analysis is performed on the basis of the way the formal pitch/rhythm contour integrates with grammar. No reference is made to the semantic or social function of the tone unit under the above headings—for example, whether the 'meaning' of the tone unit is to question, persuade, command, excite, and so on. The only reason for the lack of a classification here is the difficulty of demarcating and formally defining these notions. Intuitively, it is possible to interpret a tone unit's function in a certain way, but it is not possible, in the present state of study, to provide a systematic account of what it is that prompts these intuitions, or to list the functions in such a way that problems of overlap and ambiguity are avoided. A tone unit might give the impression of questioning, for example; but in a slightly different context, the same tone unit might give the impression of puzzlement, surprise, shock, excitement, or other attitudes. On a profile chart, it is not possible to anticipate research, nor is it possible to list all possible contextual influences. On the other hand, the chart does need to allow for the importance of these attitudes, in the evaluation of speech. A box has therefore been provided, headed *Functions*, in which might be listed any social or attitudinal contexts in which P seems to be using tone units in a distinctive way. An ad hoc label would be written in on the left side of the box, and the number of occasions when its application is observed in the data would be tallied in the usual way.

For example, a common early development in children is the use of a tone unit with a high (and usually rising) pitch range to express a set of attitudes to do with query, puzzlement etc. This is considered to be an important factor in language development, as it shows that the child is beginning to be aware of the concept of 'question'—though at this point, he lacks any grammatical structure for its expression. These 'intonational questions' are not therefore 'questions' in a grammatical sense—they would not, for example, be profiled as *Questions* on the LARSP chart (cf. 2.7.4). Nor are they always clearly questioning in attitude. But whenever high rising pitch range is interpreted in this way, T might wish to indicate the development, as a sign of progress in P—and this could easily be done by writing in *questioning,* or some such label, in the Functions box, and indicating the extent of its use in the sample. Other labels commonly encountered at an early age include: playful, demanding, uncertain, excited, aggressive . . . ; later, we have confident, sarcastic, knowing, and many more. There is of course no guarantee that what one T means by such a label will be the same as another. You and I might have quite different intuitions as to what counts as 'playful'. All the chart does is provide T with an opportunity to note down a distinctive intonational function, which illustrates P's developing linguistic range.

Similarly, any abnormal uses of intonation can be identified, as, for example, if P seemed to be using a certain type of tone unit in an inappropriate context, as when some aphasics produce empty language in a highly confident manner, or a child uses a high rising range *without* any evident intent to question, excite etc. Also under this heading would be cases where a tone unit was being commonly used in an abnormal grammatical way—making a subordinate clause more prominent than a following main clause, for example, or having a peak of prominence on clause Subjects and never on Verbs or Objects. There are hundreds of possibilities, which will in due course need a systematic statement. For the present, such points are simply noted as they arise, as in the following example taken from a language-delayed 5-year-old:

Functions

```
Questioning   15
? Bored    8
Uses V (? doubt, uncertainty) for
    clause final    12
```

4.5.5 The total number of unproblematic tone units is given at the head of the section (under *Total*). It is difficult to predict the best size of sample (cf. 1.11.1). On the whole, a sample of about 100 tone units usually suffices to show up any interesting patterns. Some Ps, with little prosodic variability, can be safely analysed from a sample of 30 or 40 tone units.

A helpful statistic, in relating intonational and grammatical form, is the average number of words in a tone unit. To calculate this, it is simplest to draw up a table, as follows:

No. of words in tone unit	No. of examples in data	Total tone units	Total words
1	12	12	12
2	8	8	16
3	11	11	33
4	10	10	40
5	2	2	10
6	0	0	0
7...	1	1	7
		44	118

Average number of words per tone unit is therefore 118/44, i.e. 2.7. (The conversational norm for adult speech is 5 words.)

4.6* As the development of intonation coincides with the use of single-element sentences, it is normal to find variation in tone occurring before variation in tonicity. Tonal variations are therefore the second kind of phenomenon to be classified on the profile chart. *Tone* here refers to the *nuclear* tones in tone units, i.e. the maximally prominent tone. Anything distinctive relating to the other tones in a tone unit can be summarized at the bottom of the chart.

4.6.1 The first—and to many people the most difficult—thing to do is to provide an accurate transcription of the tonal variation encountered in the sample. An interlinear transcriptional method is used, because there is no way of knowing in advance what phonological use is being made of the tones. Only a detailed phonetic record provides the evidence as to whether there is any system present, and this is what an interlinear transcription can provide.

Each pair of parallel lines is assumed to contain a space representing the speaker's pitch range. The upper line represents P's maximum pitch height; the lower line represents his maximum pitch depth. On the basis of T's auditory judgement, tones are then drawn in, relative to these two extremes. An example of a normal speaker follows (it should be noted that most people speak in the lower third of their possible voice range, with only occasional departures from this norm for purposes of linguistic effect):

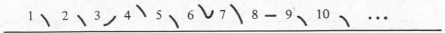

The order in which the tones are placed on the chart corresponds to the order in which they occurred in the data. Sometimes, when a close scrutiny of context is required, it proves useful to number each tone in the data, and to refer to these numbers on the chart, as follows:

In disordered prosody, one of the most notable features is the use of tones which fall completely outside the normal phonetic pattern of P's dialect. P uses a tone which does not correspond to anything in normal adult use or in the developmental stages of children acquiring the dialect (as far as is known). Such tones would therefore be called *deviant*, in our usual use of this term (cf. 2.5.1), and they are drawn in on a separate line on the profile chart (the numbering convention is here very useful, in order to locate these tones conveniently in the sample). All other tones—in other words, those within normal phonetic limits—are grouped under the heading of *variants*. As with grammatical analysis, apart from a few well-recognized types of P, the vast majority of cases in a sample are 'within normal limits'; hence more space is allowed for this category. Doubtful cases (whether normal or deviant) would be placed under *deviant* (cf. 1.9).

Some examples of transcriptions taken from Ps whose prosody was a source of concern are given below. In the first example, we see a severely delayed (ESN(S)) 10-year-old, whose tonal ability is restricted to low falling tones and a few low level tones:

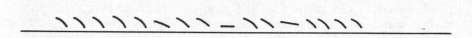

To continue the transcription, in such a case, would have added nothing: a short sample suffices.

In the next example, we have a more varied intonational picture, but one which is still very restricted, in relation to the range of possible tones in English. The child was four, and so should have been able to use all the main nuclear tones. In fact, there are no complex tones, and only high rising tones. A longer sample would be necessary for a true picture here.

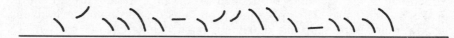

The next example shows a somewhat exaggerated pattern of tones: P is using the whole of his pitch range, and sounding excited and (for want of a better term) 'squeaky'. At times, his rising tones go outside of his normal pitch register, and he switches into falsetto (indicated by F in the transcription). His low tones go very low at times, and a creaky phonation occurs (indicated by C in the transcription). Neither the falsetto nor the creaky voice are deviant qualities, for this accent; it is the frequency of use, and the inappropriateness of these qualities which is abnormal.

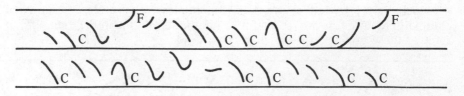

All the tones in the above examples are recognizably falling, rising, and so on; they may display peculiarities of pitch range (narrowing, widening) and phonation type, but there is nothing deviant about these pitch patterns. The following transcription, taken from a dysarthric adult, looks very different:

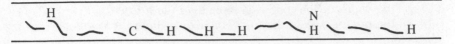

Here, there are many tones which are plainly unstable, as is evidenced by the idiosyncratic shapes of some of the pitch movements, the greater randomness of pattern, and the use of abnormal voice qualities (N stands for a nasal quality, H for a hoarse quality).

4.6.2 Once a transcription has been made, it is usually possible to see the general character of a prosodic difficulty without further analysis. On the other hand, a statistical summary of the findings can be valuable in the assessment of progress, and sometimes brings to light previously unnoticed factors (cf. 3.16). The summary matrix is organized along developmental lines, the order of emergence of the main nuclear tones being listed vertically The contrast between level (‟) and falling (`) tones usually emerges first, at around 9 months (the level tone often being associated with ritual and play situations, such as the well-known *all-gone*, often 'chanted' by parents at around this age). Next, a rising tone (´) develops, at around a year (often associated with contexts of query, surprise, delight—for example, at finding something). At about 1;3 (one year, three months), falling-rising tones (ˆ) come to be used (often associated with contexts of praise, maternal intonations of achievement, as in *good bôy*/, often using this tone). A little later, falling-rising tones (ˇ) are used (usually in the context of warning, uncertainty as to outcome, etc.—the fall-rise being a common 'danger' signal in parents' speech, as in *nŏ*/, *look ŏut*/). Compound tones (symbolized by C), by definition contain two elements which occur on different words (occasionally, on different morphemes within a word). They do not therefore occur until the emergence of multiword tone units, at or around 1;6, e.g. *dàddy thére*/. Lastly, there has to be a line available for unclear tones (?). For a variety of reasons, partly to do with analytical ability, partly with recording quality, and partly with interference from other aspects of P's disability, certainty about the direction of a nuclear tone may not be possible—and here the bottom line proves to be most convenient.

It will already be clear, from the above examples, that a wide variety of phonetic forms are used as realizations of the language's nuclear tones. The horizontal dimension of the summary matrix provides an indication of the main phonetic variations found. First of all, the most frequently occurring phonetic variant of a tone in the sample of data is identified, and referred to as the 'unmarked' or 'neutral' form, for that sample. Examples of this form are placed under the heading Ø, on the right-hand side of the matrix. The other columns, reading from right to left, summarize any distinctive phonetic variations in the use of a tone, as follows:

"   the tone is produced with extra stress;

↑   the tone has a high starting point, compared with the norm;

?↑   the tone's starting point seems higher than normal, but it is not entirely clear;

↓   the tone has a low starting point, compared with the norm;

W   the width of the tone is greater than the norm;

N   the pitch-range of the tone is narrower than the norm.

Other then refers to tones which have any other kinds of phonetic distinctiveness, such as the abnormal voice qualities already noted, or any combinations of the above phonetic variations (such as high narrow, wide extra stress).

We can illustrate the set of possibilities by taking a falling tone, and showing how one would move from its transcription to the appropriate cell on the summary matrix. The transcription produced the following range of tones:

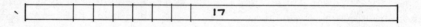

It is evident that a mid-to-low tone is the norm, in this case. All instances of this form are counted, and the number transferred to the Ø column, opposite.

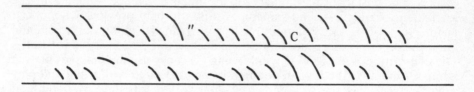

Each of the remaining tones is then judged in relation to this norm, as follows:

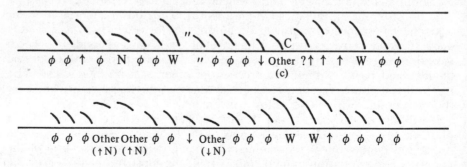

Each category is then counted, and the totals transferred to the relevant column along the falling-tone line, as follows:

(It is not always necessary to spell out the categories under *Other.*)

Three methodological points should be noted:

(a) The contrasts *N* and *W* cannot by definition apply to level tone.

(b) The complex tones ˇ and ˆ are not subclassified in terms of their phonetic types, other than the gross distinctions recognized above. For example, the normal phonetic form of the fall-rise in English is ‾ᴠ‾. A 'widened' version of this tone could therefore be any of the following:

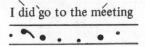

All of these would be counted under *W*, in the profile procedure. Other kinds of complex tone (such as rise-fall-rise) are considered to be variants of the two basic types recognized on the chart: a rise-fall-rise is seen as a variant of fall-rise; a fall-rise-fall as a variant of rise-fall; and so on.

(c) Similarly, variations in compound tones are not subclassified. The category, first of all, subsumes fall-plus-rise, rise-plus-fall, and permitted variants thereof (such as rise-fall-plus-rise). The normal phonetic form for, say, a fall-plus-rise is a smooth contour forming a 'trough', as in:

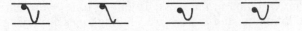

Phonetic variations in this form might thus include: $\uparrow` + ´$, $` + \uparrow ´$, $` + N´$, $\uparrow W` + ´$, $N` + N´$, and so on. These are placed under the appropriate category without any further classification. For example, all of the following are placed under *W:*

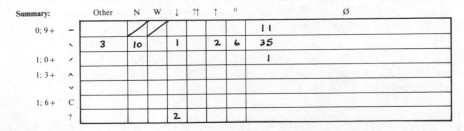

4.6.3 It should now be possible to make an initial assessment of prosodic disability using the summary matrix, which—because of its developmental perspective—can then be a source of suggestions for remediation. The following summary, for instance, presents a fairly straightforward case of prosodic delay:

Summary:		Other	N	W	↓	?↑	↑	‖		∅
0; 9 +	–		⟋⟋					I I		
	＼	3	10		I	2	6	35		
1; 0 +	／							I		
1; 3 +	^									
	˅									
1; 6 +	C									
	?			2						

In this sample, there were 11 instances of a level tone, all at about the same pitch level and loudness (so there are no grounds for using the other cells along the line). There were 57 falling tones in the sample, 35 of which were of the same phonetic type, and thus taken as a norm. (Reference to the transcriptional lines would show what phonetic form was involved.) Of the remainder, 6 were falling tones identical to the norm apart from an extra degree of stress; 2 were falling tones identical in loudness to the norm, but having a high starting point; 1 falling tone had a distinctively low starting point, but no variation in loudness; 10 falling tones were narrowed, with no variation in loudness; and there were 3 falling tones displaying other prosodic characteristics. In addition, there was a single example of a rising tone in the sample, and 2 cases where it was unclear which tone was involved (due to the low starting-point, which had made it unclear whether the tones were falling or level).

A somewhat more advanced level of ability is presented in the next summary (note especially the apparent contrast between fall and high fall, rise and high rise):

Summary:		Other	N	W	↓	?↑	↑	‖	∅
0;9+	−		╱	╱					3
	＼		2				11		31
1;0+	／						10		16
1;3+	∧								
	∨								1
1;6+	C								
	?								8

A highly abnormal development is encountered in the next summary:

Summary:		Other	N	W	↓	?↑	↑	‖	∅
0;9+	−		╱	╱					2
	＼					3	1		3
1;0+	／	6		3			11		8
1;3+	∧								
	∨			1			7	2	24
1;6+	C								
	?								

It would seem as if the falling-rising tone has taken over some of the functions of the falling tone (cf. also 4.9).

4.6.3 It should also be recognized that P may be making a tentative phonological use of phonetic distinctions which are not those of the normal adult language. Take the following tonal profile, for example:

Summary:	Other	N	W	↓	?↑	↑	‖	∅
0; 9+ −		⧄	⧄				7	
`				11	3	21	40	
1; 0+ ´							4	
1; 3+ ˄								
˅								
1; 6+ C								
?								

There is some evidence here of a contrast in pitch range, with a clear norm, and two departures from this norm—high and low. Whether or not these distinctions are contrastive phonologically would only emerge from an examination of the contexts in which the phonetic forms are used. It might be, for example, that the high falling tones are always used in contexts of surprise, and the low in contexts of routine activity. At least there is now a testable hypothesis to work with, and the possibility of a more precise understanding of the nature of P's condition.

4.7* The third main section of the profile chart deals with *tonicity*, the placement within a tone unit of its nuclear tone. As with tone unit identification, we have to allow for unclear cases. Even if a tone unit has been unambiguously identified, there may still be uncertainty over its internal structure or how to interpret it. Three main types of difficulty are routinely encountered:

(a) Indeterminate tonicity occurs when, within a complete tone unit, the placement of the nuclear tone (whether simple, complex or compound) is unclear. Usually, this is because there is competition between two words in the tone unit for the assignment of nucleus: sometimes one sounds prominent, sometimes the other. Under such circumstances, it is best to avoid making a decision.

(b) Under the heading of *stereotyped* tonicity would be included any case where the placement of the nuclear tone is fixed. There may or may not be other kinds of prosodic variation in the tone unit. A clear example of stereotyped tonicity occurs in the prosodic pattern of limericks, or in reciting one's tables; idioms, too, usually have a fixed tonicity pattern ('it's raining cats and *dogs*', never '*cats* and dogs'). A stereotyped tonicity generally coincides with stereotyping elsewhere—often the tone-unit structure as a whole is stereotyped, as is the choice of nuclear tone, and the underlying grammatical pattern.

(c) It is often the case that P *imitates* the tonicity pattern of T's stimulus, and the resulting pattern ought therefore to be considered separately. For example, one P who had never used contrastive tonicity in his spontaneous speech was heard to produce the following:

T	was the cát 'hurt/ or the dòg 'hurt/
P	'cat hùrt/
T	nó/
	the ''dòg was 'hurt/
P	dòg 'hurt/

Given the clear stimulus, it would be premature to assume that P was able to control the contrastivity normally associated with bringing the tone forward in the sentence in this way. All such cases of apparent imitation would not be further analysed.

4.7.1 The tonicity matrix makes a primary division in terms of whether the nuclear tone falls on the last item in a tone unit (*Final*) or precedes this item (*Non-Final*). A distinction is then drawn between whether the item in question is a lexical item (*table, chair, run, nice. . .*) or a grammatical item (*in, is, to, the. . .*). The reason for distinguishing between grammatical and lexical terms, with respect to tonic placement, is to do with both assessment and remediation. Because grammatical items belong to relatively small and fixed sets of words (the system of pronouns, of articles, of prepositions etc.), the nature of the contrast imposed when one of these words carries the nuclear tone is wholly different from that imposed when lexical items are given the nuclear tone. If I say 'Put it *near* John', there is very little to contrast *near* with—close to or far away from, but not much more. On the other hand, if I say 'Put it near *John*', there could be an indefinite number of contrasts, depending on the number of people or objects in the vicinity. A P who has difficulty with the contrastivity on grammatical items will therefore require a somewhat different kind of therapy than one who has difficulty with the contrastivity on lexical items. The two are consequently kept distinct on the profile chart, for the analysis of simple tones. (The more complex tones, such as fall-plus-rise and rise-plus-fall, are not subdivided in this way, as they are insufficiently frequently used to warrant it.)

Within each tone unit, then, the item carrying the nuclear tone is identified as either grammatical or lexical. Doubtful cases are assigned to the *lexical* category (as this makes fewer assumptions about the type of item involved). If the item is final in the tone unit, it is assigned to the right-hand section of the matrix; if it is nonfinal, it is assigned to the left-hand section. (A tone-unit consisting of a single item is taken as final.) A decision is then made as to whether P's tonic placement is appropriate or not, in relation to the grammatical structure of his utterance and what he was thought to be wanting to say. If his tonic placement is correct and appropriate, a mark is placed under the column headed by $\sqrt{}$. If it is not, the mark goes into the column headed by X.

Each of these possibilities is illustrated in the following set of examples (all with falling nuclear tones):

he '*spoke to the màn*/   Lexical item, Final, Appropriate
'*cat hùrt*/ (the example in 4.7 above)   Lexical item, Final, Inappropriate
'*put it ìn*/   Grammatical item, Final, Appropriate
that's '*where I* '*went tò*/   Grammatical item, Final, Inappropriate
the dòg's '*hurt*/ (i.e. not the cat)   Lexical item, Nonfinal, Appropriate
the màn's '*running*/ (where there is only a man in the picture)   Lexical item, Nonfinal, Inappropriate
'*put it ìn the* '*box*/ (i.e. not under)   Grammatical item, Nonfinal, Appropriate
'*put ìt in the* '*box*/   Grammatical item, Nonfinal, Inappropriate

It should be noted that there may be two reasons for the inappropriate placement of the nuclear tone: it may simply be incorrect, in the sense of 'never possible', as when the sentence *it's raining* is pronounced with tonic *it* (because *it* is empty of meaning, there could be no case where a tonic contrast would be meaningful); or the tonic placement may be possible, but misleading, as when P draws attention to a word without intending to (as in the *man running* example above). These two possibilities are not distinguished on the profile chart, but they must always be borne in mind when interpreting the figures.

In normal adult conversation, about 90 per cent of the nuclear tones fall on the last lexical item in a tone unit. A normal adult profile of tonicity would therefore look something like this:

	Non Final		Final	
Simple	✓	×	✓	×
Lexical	10		40	
Grammatical	3		5	

By contrast, the following illustrate two cases of disability:

	Non Final		Final	
Simple	✓	×	✓	×
Lexical			20	10
Grammatical			5	15

This is a common pattern in language delay. P has not learned to use tonicity contrastively, and mechanically places the nuclear tone on the final item in the tone unit, regardless of its appropriateness.

	Non Final		Final	
Simple	✓	×	✓	×
Lexical	4	13	30	3
Grammatical	5	2	10	0

Here, the picture is more complex. P is evidently bringing his nuclear tones forward in the tone unit, but has not learned the rules governing their use. He makes more errors with lexical items, suggesting that his problem is more to do with the semantics of what he is saying than with the grammar.

4.7.2 The compound tones are not given such a detailed statement, because of their infrequency. As a first approximation, the chart provides space only for an indication of where in the tone unit the 2 elements of the compound are to be located. In the right-hand column, the tonic elements are Nonfinal and Final respectively (NF + F); in the left-hand column, they are both on Nonfinal items (NF + NF). For example:

NF+F: *he'll be hère tomórrow/*
NF+F: *'John sàid he'd cóme/*

NF+NF: *whère are you góing to'morrow/*
NF+NF: *pùt a cóin in 'will you/*

These would be marked on the chart as follows:

Complex	NF + NF \ + ⁄ 2	NF + F \ + ⁄ 2

4.8 The remaining section of the PROP chart allows for a brief note of any *Other* features of prosodic interest in the data. It is recognized that there is space for only a token mention, and that if these other features were at all numerous, it would be necessary to handle them on a supplementary page. Four categories are given:

(a) Tone unit pitch refers to other pitch patterns in the tone unit apart from those discussed above. For example, the pitch levels of the tones other than the nuclear tone may be of interest, as may the overall tonal configuration which constitutes the *head* of the tone unit. The following example illustrates an abnormal head pattern:

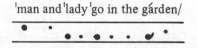

The sudden pitch drop after the first stressed item was typical of this P, and gave a strange (and highly distracting) chant effect to the beginning of his sentences. The point would have been summarized under Other, using some convenient notation or shorthand account.

(b) Tone unit other refers to any prosodic patterns *other than pitch* which might affect the character of a tone unit—such as variations in the loudness, speed, rhythm or pauses used. One aphasic P would always give the first part of a sentence extra loudness and speed, which would then tail away rapidly. A child P would pause erratically in attempting to use Subjects in clauses. These are the kinds of points which would be summarized in this section—again, using some convenient ad hoc notation.

(c) Under the heading *Prosodic features (TU+)* are included any prosodic features (including pitch) which extend over a stretch of utterance longer than a tone unit. For example, P might say several sentences in a single high pitch range, with many tone units affected. Or a certain rhythm, loudness or speed might be given to a tone unit sequence. The particular combination of variables would be noted, along with an indication of their extent, e.g.

'high/fast/loud 4'—in other words, a sequence of 4 tone units was produced in a high, fast and loud manner.

(*d*) Any other nonsegmental phonological characteristics of speech are summarized under the heading of *paralinguistic features*. These are counted separately, whether they occur within or across tone units. Examples of such tones of voice include whisper, breathy, giggle, falsetto, labialized, and many other 'voices' which P might adopt in a role play situation.

4.9* An illustration of the whole PROP procedure now follows, beginning with the transcription, and continuing with the profiling and subsequent interpretation. The case is a 9-year-old language-delayed child, who presented with several problems of attention span and short-term memory, a number of difficulties in clause and phrase structure, and a fairly marked nonfluency. T's prosody is also transcribed, but not formally analysed.

		Tone unit	Tone	Tonicity
P	and erm –	Incomplete	–	–
	and erm –	Incomplete	–	–
	I 'I .	Incomplete	–	–
	I 'I wañt .	Incomplete	–	–
	I wañt .	Incomplete	–	–
	erm a bíngo/	Phrase	´Ø	Final lexical √
	gámc/	Word	´Ø	Final lexical √
T	a whát/			
P	a ''bìngo/	Phrase	`''	Final lexical √
T	bìngo/			
P	yèah/	Word	`Ø	Final lexical √
T	m̀/			
P	ha .'have be 'lots of mòney . 'in/	Clause	`Ø	Nonfinal lexical √
T	it has 'lots of ↑ mòney in/			
P	yèah/	Word	`Ø	Final lexical √
T	dóes it/			
P	and –	Incomplete	–	–
	and erm .	Incomplete	–	–
	[ə] we 'have a (*4 sýlls*)/.	Indeterminate	´Ø	Indeterminate
	and erm . a 'set dĭce/	Phrase	`Ø	Final lexical √
	and 'guess which nŭmber/ –	Clause	`Ø	Final lexical √
	and erm .	Incomplete	–	–
	and erm –	Incomplete	–	–
	[a] 'you [a] 'you mŏve/	Cl–	`Ø	Final lexical √
	abouꞆ –– [a] óne or/	Cl–	´Ø	Nonfinal lexical √
	twó or/	Cl–	´Ø	Nonfinal lexical √
	tén/	Word	´Ø	Final lexical √
	tíme/	Word	´Ø	Final lexical √
T	m̀/			
P	and erm .	Incomplete	–	–
	[a] 'when . [a wə a]	Incomplete	–	–
	'when you 'get . s . 'something – 'on the mǎn/	Clause	`Ø	Final lexical √

	[ə] we [ə] 'have to ↑ read thăt/	Clause	ˋØ	Final grammatical √
	[ə] be 'what 'this săy/	Cl+	ˋØ	Final lexical √
T	what ìs it/			
	a cărd/ –			
P	nò/	Word	ˋØ	Final lexical √
	[ə] be 'like erm –––			
	[ə] be 'like a ↑ bòok or 'something/	Clause	ˋ ↑	Nonfinal lexical √
T	m̌/			
P	and erm – [əə]	Incomplete	–	–
	whăt 'this 'say/ ––	Clause	ˉØ	Nonfinal grammatical
	hów/ –	Word	´Ø	Final grammatical √
	hów/	Word	´Ø	Final grammatical √
	mǎny/ .	Word	ˋØ	Final grammatical √
	tǐme/	Word	ˋØ	Final lexical √
	are 'you have to 'move tèn/	Cl–	ˋØ	Final lexical √
T	m̀/			
	I sée/ .			
P	and erm .	Incomplete	–	–
	[ə] gǔess/ –	Word	ˋØ	Final lexical √
	and erm –	Incomplete	–	–
	'after 'you . 'having 'got			
	a prǐze/ –	Clause	ˋØ	Final lexical √
	[ə] 'you –	Incomplete	–	–
	[ə] 'you căn/ –	Cl–	ˋØ	Final grammatical √
	mǒve/	Word	ˋØ	Final lexical √
	a'bout ↑ ten ↑ tìme/	Phrase	ˋ ↑	Final lexical √
T	I sèe/ ––			
	and 'who's 'going to bùy this 'for you/––			
P	Nàn is/	Clause	ˋØ	Nonfinal lexical √

This is only a short extract, but it should suffice to illustrate the principles involved. The next step is to transfer the analysis to the profile chart (see p. 137).

An analysis of this sample shows Ian's tone unit and tonal systems to be seriously disturbed. His nonfluency often disrupts his rhythm, and prompts the analysis of many fragments as separate but incomplete tone units. His complete tone units display an erratic and deviant relationship to grammar, as is indicated mainly by the high figure for *Word* and *Cl-*. His nuclear tones are predominantly rising or falling-rising, giving a permanently dubious, cautious tone of voice to his speech, and one which leads to misunderstanding. By ending so many utterances with rising-type tones, it is never clear whether Ian has stopped talking and is waiting for a reply, or whether he is about to continue, after a nonfluent pause. His use of rises and fall-rises in utterance-final position breaks a major semantic expectancy for this dialect, and also does not correspond to what we would expect in normal language acquisition.

An important remedial goal is thus to restore or provide (there was no record kept as to how longstanding a problem this had been) a balanced tonal system and a rhythmically more coherent tone-unit structure. It would be

Prosody Profile (PROP)

Name	Ian J.	Duration	1 min. 30 secs.
Age	9	Sample date 10.4.80	Type Free conversation

Tone Unit (0; 9+)

Total **30**   Average words **2·7**

Structures

Incomplete	15	Indeterminate	1	Stereotyped	Imitation
Clause	8			**Functions**	
Phrase	4				
Word	12			√ sentence final	
Other Cl+	1				
Cl−	5				

Tone (0; 9+)

Data Variants ∕ ∕ ∖ ∖ ∖ ∖ ∨ ∨ ∨ ∕ ∕ ∕ ∕ ∨ ∨ ∨ ∖ − ∕ ∕ ∨ ∨
∖ ∨ ∨ ∨ ∨ ∖ ∖

Deviant

Summary:		Other	N	W	↓	?↑	↑	‖	Ø
0; 9+	−								1
	＼					2	1		6
1; 0+	∕								9
1; 3+	∧								
	∨								12
1; 6+	C								
	?								

Tonicity (1; 6+)

	Indeterminate	Stereotyped	Imitation

	Non Final		Final	
Simple	√	×	√	×
Lexical	5		19	
Grammatical	1		5	
Complex	NF+NF		NF+F	

Other

Tone unit pitch		Prosodic features (TU+)	
Tone unit other	3	Paraling features	

important to tie in such therapy with ongoing work on grammar and attention. For example, if T decided to introduce a rising-tone/falling-tone sequence, to teach the idea of 'nonfinal'/'final', it would be important (a) to ensure that this antithesis was introduced on grammatical structures well within Ian's grasp (avoiding, for example, tense contrasts, which still at times elude him), and (b) to maintain a clear cognitive relationship between language and task (e.g. by presenting a 2-element action sequence with a clear beginning and end, thus not motivating the open-ended narrative which feeds Ian's inattention). *The 'man 'kicks the ↑ báll/ and 'scores a ↓ gòal/* would be an example of such a determinate sequence (along with appropriate phonetic reinforcement of the contrast, using pitch range).

5 PRISM

5.1* Any attempt at a semantic profile chart, given our limited theoretical and empirical knowledge of the way linguistic meaning is structured and acquired, is full of major pitfalls. It is certainly not possible to construct a chart which could claim to be as principled as those discussed elsewhere in this book. On the other hand, semantic problems do play a significant role in the assessment and remediation of many child and adult Ps, and some systematic way of focusing T's attention on the nature of these problems is urgently needed. The procedure known as PRISM (*'Profile in Semantics'*) is a first attempt towards this goal. It has been a useful tool in organizing ideas about semantic disability and remediation, even though it raises several problems for which arbitrary solutions have had to be devised, in order to promote consistency of use.

5.2 There are two main features to note about the PRISM procedure. Firstly, it is presented as a combination of two subprocedures—one dealing with the relationship between semantics and grammar (PRISM-G), the other with the relationship between semantics and lexicon (PRISM-L). It is important to stress the importance of having both a grammatical and a lexical dimension for semantic analysis. While most people identify semantic analysis with vocabulary (or lexicon), it must not be forgotten that the meaning of a word is largely dependent on the context in which it is used, and that therefore the word's role in a sentence needs to be taken into account. Notions such as 'actor', 'action' and 'location' provide an essential alternative dimension of analysis to the grammatical concepts of Subject, Verb, Adverbial etc. discussed in Chapter 2. PRISM-G is essentially a descriptive framework for the analysis of the meanings conveyed by the different grammatical elements of a sentence. It is a 3-page chart, constructed along similar lines to LARSP, but with the patterns defined according to semantic (as opposed to syntactic or morphological) criteria.

Secondly, the most noticeable characteristic of the procedure is the size of the PRISM-L component—16 pages, instead of the 1 or 2 typical of other profiles. The reason for the chart's greater size is the extent of the vocabulary which it has to incorporate. Phonological and grammatical procedures are relatively straightforward, in that they have to deal with only 100 or so variables; it is therefore reasonable to expect that short samples of connected speech will be fairly representative (apart from in certain well-recognized situations), and that it will be possible to summarize the use of these variables in a page or two. But the commonly-occurring 'domestic' vocabulary of daily life runs into several thousand lexical items. It is obvious that a sense of P's lexical range will not be established from a short sample, nor can it be usefully organized into a couple of pages. The primary characteristic of PRISM-L, accordingly, is its extensive inventory of lexical fields, into which (in principle) the whole of P's vocabulary can be incorporated. The detailed classification is needed in order to provide a discriminating assessment of P's lexical range, and to identify lexical areas for remediation. To meet these criteria, a chart of several pages is unavoidable.

5.3 Before outlining the descriptive frameworks, certain theoretical considerations need to be briefly reviewed:

(a)* Lexical terminology needs to be clearly distinguished from grammatical, if the discussion of disability is to be unambiguous. The term *word* is a recognized part of grammatical metalanguage, and hence a different term is needed to discuss the minimal units of vocabulary. In the present book, the terms *lexical item* and *lexeme* are used (interchangeably) to refer to these minimal units—in other words, the items which would be listed as head-words in a dictionary. It should be noted that grammatical variants are ignored in specifying lexemes: for example, *walk, walks, walking, walked* are all variants of the same lexeme WALK (conventionally printed in small capitals); *is, are, am, be, been, was, were* are all variants of the lexeme BE; and so on. Also, it should be noted that some lexical items may consist of more than one word, e.g. *spick and span, kick the bucket* ('die') (and all idioms), *switch on* (and all phrasal verbs), *too many cooks spoil the broth* (and all proverbs).

(b) While the PRISM-L procedure is presented as an inventory of lexical fields, it must be remembered that this is only the first step in the investigation of P's semantic system. The lexicon of a language is *not* an inventory, but a system of contrasts. The business of lexical analysis is to identify the types of contrast which interrelate the lexical items in a language—contrasts such as sameness of meaning, oppositeness of meaning, and so on. These contrasts can not usually be established on the basis of a profile analysis of a sample of spontaneous speech, however; they need to be elicited in structured situations (see further, 5.7.7). On the other hand, unless one has some units of vocabulary with which to operate, it is impossible to carry out the more advanced, structured work. The aim of PRISM-L, therefore, is to provide an initial classification of lexical items, which can provide the motivation for a more principled investigation of P's semantic system than would otherwise be possible.

(c)* In its emphasis on vocabulary (in the present case, on English), the business of semantic analysis must be rigorously distinguished from the concerns of cognitive studies. While cognitive problems are often the reasons for the failure of P to develop an adequate lexical system, any statement of lexical difficulty can and should be made, in the first instance, independently of cognitive considerations. It is possible to have semantic disability within an otherwise intact cognitive ability, which illustrates the need to keep the distinction clear.

(d)* Similarly, the various units and categories presented on the PRISM charts are 'neutral' in respect to the question of production or comprehension. One may use PRISM, as with any profile, either as a guide to production or as a guide to comprehension of the lexical items and sentence patterns it

contains. Unless one introduces a specific convention, marking a specific lexical item or sentence pattern onto the charts says nothing about whether P has understood it: it simply indicates that he has used the item/pattern (if the study is of his expressive language), or had the item/pattern used to him (if the study is of his receptive language). It is a separate analytical decision to say how efficiently these items/patterns have been processed by P, whether some kind of 'comprehension problem' is involved.

5.4 The PRISM-L chart consists of 16 pages, arranged in the following manner:

page 1 contains a summary of the data samples used, including a brief quantitative statement (see further, 5.7.9);
page 2 contains an inventory of *minor* lexical items (see further, 5.6);
page 3 contains a quantitative summary of the *major* lexical items listed on pages 4 to 15 (see further, 5.7.6);
pages 4 to 15 contain a classification of lexical items in terms of the main semantic fields in which they occur (see further, 5.7);
page 16 contains sections in which can be recorded observations about P's systematic use of lexemes (see further, 5.7.7).

5.4.1 The input to the PRISM-L analysis is a transcription of P's language, in either phonological or orthographic form. Each sentence is taken, and its constituent lexical items identified, as in the following examples:

Words	*the*	*man*	*is*	*going*	*to*	*town*		
Lexemes	THE	MAN	BE	GO	TO	TOWN		
Words	*he*	*sat*	*down*	*on*	*his*	*chair*		
Lexemes	HE	SIT	DOWN	ON	HE	CHAIR		
Words	*I*	*had*	*asked*	*him*	*for*	*the*	*best*	*eggs*
Lexemes	I	HAVE	ASK	HE	FOR	THE	GOOD	EGG

If there is doubt as to the assignment of a word to a lexeme, the policy is to underanalyse—that is, *not* to conflate words under the same lexeme. For example, it might not be clear, in certain circumstances, whether a sequence such as *ask for* was to be considered one lexeme or two (in grammatical terms, is it a phrasal verb or not?). In such cases, the words would be taken as separate items, and entered onto the PRISM chart accordingly.

5.5 It should be plain, from just these examples, that the items in a sentence are of several different types. Some items are evidently 'full' of meaning, in the sense that it is usually possible to make a statement about the role of an item in relation to the external world—MAN, GO, TOWN, CHAIR etc. Others have less of an evident relationship to the external world, and are more concerned with the way in which items relate to each other grammatically—THE, BE, TO, etc. The PRISM-L procedure assumes that *all* items need to be investigated, from a semantic point of view, but recognizes that these two general types will pose different questions for assessment, and require different strategies in remediation. A distinction is therefore introduced at the outset, between *major* and *minor* lexical items. Major items correspond to the so-called 'content' or 'lexical' words of traditional approaches—the indefinitely large set of items which categorize our actions, entities, perceptions etc. Minor items include the so-called 'function' or 'grammatical' words of traditional approaches—the small, closed sets of items which express grammatical relationships; but certain other items, which are semantically unproductive, are also included under this heading.

5.6 Page 2 of the procedure provides a classification of minor lexical items. The page is divided into 4 main sections:

(i) stretches of utterance whose lexical status it is impossible to analyse;
(ii) lexical items whose function seems primarily *social,* in that their role is to maintain a satisfactory conversational relationship between speaker and hearer;
(iii) lexical items whose function is primarily *relational,* in the sense that their role is the expression of grammatical notions within sentences;
(iv) items whose role is to 'fill the gap', when specific major or minor lexical items are unavailable to P (as in the classical 'word-finding' problems); this section is headed *avoidance.*

These sections are arranged on page 2 as follows:

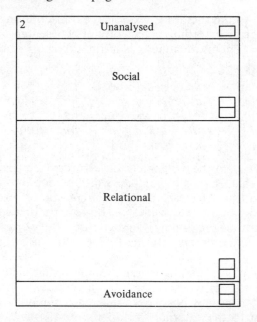

5.6.1 Under the heading of Unanalysed are placed all cases where it is not possible to be sure what lexical item P is using—or whether any lexical item is there at all. This category thus includes cases of Unintelligibility, for whatever reason; Ambiguity, where it is not possible to say what meaning an item has, and thus under which category it should go (whether major or minor, or under which subcategory of major or minor); and Symbolic Noise, where P's mimicking of real-world events is noted, but without further classification. A category of Other is provided for any further cases of uncertain analysis which might be encountered. These categories are laid out as follows:

Unanalysed	Unintelligible	Ambiguous	Symbolic Noise	Other	Totals

Obtaining an accurate impression of unintelligible items is often not easy. There is little problem when part of an utterance is plainly a single obscure lexical item, as in *he got a glogle;* but when a whole stretch of utterance is affected by phonological uncertainty, nonfluency and other such factors, it is often not possible to do more than give an approximate indication of the number of lexical items affected.

The total number of unanalysed items is noted in the box on the right-hand side of the section, and then transferred to the summary on page 1, for comparison with other totals (see further, 5.7.9).

5.6.2 Five subcategories are recognized under the heading of *social* items. The first two subcategories are best explained together.

(a) and *(b) Spontaneous and Response*   Spontaneous items are those minor sentences (cf. 2.7) introduced into the conversation by P, without any dependency on a T stimulus. Examples include *hello, oh!, gosh!* Response items are those minor sentences which P uses primarily as a response to a T stimulus, such as *yes, no* or *m* in reply to questions. Other examples include *thanks, pardon, well.* It should be noted that some items may be either spontaneous or response, depending on context; for example, P may use *yes* to answer questions, but also use it spontaneously (e.g. saying it to herself while playing with toys). The set of social spontaneous and response items used by one P in a 30-minute sample was as follows:

Spontaneous	Response	
hello 2	yes 15	pardon 1
yes 2	yeah 7	oh 2
ah 3	no 25	thank you 2
oops 1	m 6	

(Here, and throughout this chapter, the marking convention is illustrated as follows: *hullo* ‖ means that *hullo* has been used twice.)

(c) Stereotypes   These are cases where there are grounds for taking a multiword string as a single lexical unit, lacking any productive internal structure. Examples include proverbs, nursery rhyme extracts, catch phrases, titles of books, and the whole range of 'favourite' or 'automatic' phrases P might use. An example from an adult (aphasic) sample was as follows:

Stereotype	laughed like a drain 3
beg pardon 10	not to worry 2
very nicely 6	Tom Brown's Days 1
oh dear me 16	
see what I mean 8	
13 Letchworth Drive 2	

(d) Comment Under this heading is included the restricted range of clauses whose function is parenthetic or marginal to the meaning and structure of the sentence, such as *you see, you know, mind you, I mean, the trouble is, to be honest* etc. There are no grounds in these cases for a lexical analysis in terms of *you + know, I + mean,* and so on, and they are classified here as if they were single items. Tag questions, which have certain similarities to these comment clauses, are listed under *interrogatives* further down page 2 (see 5.6.3 (d)).

(e) Proper names are quite different semantically from all other lexical items in language, and need to be taken separately. An example from a child sample is as follows:

Proper N	Reading 1
mummy 3	Butlins 1
nan 1	
daddy 5	
Tony 1	
Mrs Jackson 2	

(f) A category of *Other* has to be recognized, as it is likely that, as more Ps come to be analysed, items will be encountered which do not fit readily into the above 5 categories.

The layout of the Social Minor section of the chart is therefore as follows:

Spontaneous	Response
Stereotype	Comment
Proper N	Other

5.6.3 *Relational* items are those whose primary function is grammatical, i.e. they operate as part of a closed system of contrasts, such as the articles, pronouns and auxiliary verbs. On the LARSP chart, one notes the total number of items belonging to each of these systems, but no reference is made to the range of individual items used within a system—for example, 'Pron 27' does not indicate whether the pronouns used were *I, you, mine, she,* or whatever. It is the lexical range of each system which the relational section of the PRISM chart is designed to display. On the whole, grammatical terms are used as category labels—partly to enable a convenient cross-reference to be made to the LARSP chart, but also because there is no widely-agreed semantic terminology for handling the meanings involved under each heading. Eight subcategories are recognized:

(a) Pronominal All items with direct person or object reference are placed under this heading. The conventional distinction between 1st, 2nd and 3rd person pronouns is used, but these notions are interpreted semantically. Under 1st person, for example, would be included *I, my, mine, we, our, ours, myself, ourselves, us, one* (in certain contexts), and so on—but not if one of these items were given a special use (as when *we* refers to a 3rd person, e.g. therapist about consultant: *we're in a bad mood today*). *This, that, these, those, it* and *they* (in certain contexts), along with their variants, are the main object-reference items in English, and these are counted separately, using the label demonstrative *(Dem)*. The definite and indefinite articles, because of their close grammatical and semantic links with these items, are also included in this column (under *Art*). Under *Other* would be placed items where reference is nonspecific or ambiguous, as in certain uses of *one, we, you* (e.g. *you down here, turn right . . .*), and so on. An example of the use of this category taken from a language-delayed 4-year-old whose pronoun use was fairly advanced, is as follows:

Pronominal								
1	I 3	my 8	me 12		Dem	that 17	they 7	It 8	its 2
2	you 8	your 10			Art	a 11	the 5
3	he 6	she 2	her 2		Other		
	they 1	them 1					

This was a single sample of only 15 minutes, so the gaps may be fortuitous; subsequent observation would confirm this, or alternatively indicate whether there may be a genuine lexico-grammatical weakness (e.g. in the 1st person 'plural' items).

(b) Prepositional This category provides a lexical breakdown of the range of prepositions in English, classified in terms of their primary semantic function—locative *(Loc)* (e.g. *under, near*), temporal *(Temp)* (e.g. *for, since*), and *Other* (manner, e.g. *by;* cause, e.g. *because of;* etc.). It should be noted that most prepositions can be used in a variety of semantic contexts: *on*, for example, has a locative use (*on the table*), a temporal use (*on Monday*), and so on. There will also be several uncertain uses (e.g. *in uniform*), for which a category of Problems is required. Clearly idiomatic constructions, however, are taken as lexical wholes, and classified as major items below (see 5.7), e.g. *as well, on purpose, for instance*.

The following illustration of the use of the Prepositional category on page 2 of the chart is taken from the same child as in (a) above:

Prepositional				Other	of 5
Loc					like 3
in 16	to 7	into 1		Temp	
on 6	at 3			at 8 for 3	Problems
down 1	with 2			in 2	in 3
against 1				about 3	of 2

The restricted prepositional range is noteworthy, for a 4-year-old, and frequency is low, even for a 15-minute sample. Further systematic investigation of this area would seem to be warranted.

(c) Verbs whose function is primarily or purely grammatical are listed in the next section. *Be,* in all its forms, is the main item, in view of its frequency, and it is tabulated separately under 1st, 2nd and 3rd person (no distinction being made between copula and auxiliary function). *Other* verbs include the remaining auxiliaries, whether modal or other (as distinguished in LARSP: cf. 2.11.2), e.g. the various forms of *do, have, will, can, might, let;* also the pro-verb *do* (as in *Yes he does*). The use of a negative word or particle within the verb phrase (whether in full or contracted form) is given its own place on the right of the section (under *Neg*). Full forms, such as *no, not,* are counted separately under *Neg*. Contracted forms are listed along with their verbs, e.g. *isn't, won't.* A normal 2½-year-old produced the following lexical range in this column, in a short sample:

Verbal							
be 1	am 3	'm 2					
2			Other		Neg		
3	be 3	's 5	can 1		won't 3		
			did 3		can't 4		
			'll 2		not 2	no 1	
			do 3				

(d) Interrogatives include the whole range of items conventionally referred to as 'question-words', whether used in direct or indirect speech (cf. <u>where</u> *is he going, he asked* <u>where</u> *he was going*). In view of their infrequency in most clinical samples, a further semantic classification (into place, time, manner, animate, inanimate, etc.) has not been made. To give a good example of their range, therefore, the following illustration has been used, taken from the semantic analysis of *therapist* questions used in a 15-minute session with a 5-year-old language delayed child:

Interrogative	what for 2
what 31	how 6
who 10	what sort 1
what else 16	what about 3
where 9	how many 1
which 1	why 1
	whose 1

(e) Tag questions and statements are listed under the heading Tags, without further classification, e.g. *isn't he, are we, he is* (as in *he's nice, he is*). The relevance of intonation may need to be noted (rising tones for the 'questioning' sense, falling tones for the 'informing' sense).

(f) Connectives subsume the lexical items used as coordinating and subordinating conjunctions in grammar, such as *and, but, if, after*. Because of their infrequency in most samples, no further subclassification into semantic types (such as time or cause) has been made—though this could be added if required. A typical example of the use of connectives is seen in this child of 3 (who was just commencing LARSP Stage V: cf. 2.13):

Connective	
and	31
when	3
'cos	1
before	2

The frequency of *and* is noteworthy, as is the development of elementary temporal forms.

(g) For the sake of completeness, semantically 'empty' items are allowed a place on the chart, though they are strictly relevant only for the study of grammar, e.g. *it* (in such contexts as *it's raining, it was in the garden that I met him*), *there* (as in *there were lots in the shop*) and *to* (as in *I want to go, it's time to stop*).

(h) A category of Other is recognized for those relational items which do not fit clearly into any of the above-mentioned categories (such as *so,* in *I think so,* etc.).

The layout of the relational section of the chart is thus as follows:

Pronominal		
1	Dem	
2	Art	
3	Other	
Prepositional		Other
Loc	Temp	
		Problems
Verbal		
be 1	Other	Neg
2		
3		
Interrogative	Tags	
Connective		
Empty	Other	

5.6.4 We note separately, under the heading of Avoidance, the use of any lexeme whose purpose is clearly to stand in for a different lexeme, which P does not have available (for whatever reason—whether he has lost it, not yet learned it, forgotten it, etc.). Common adult aphasic examples include *whatsits, whatsisname, thingy,* and there may be idiosyncratic avoidance items.

5.6.5 The numerical summary of each section of page 2 of the chart (apart from Unanalysed) is made in terms of both Types and Tokens. It is plainly important to know whether P's totals are due to his frequent use of a small range of social/relational/avoidance items, or whether he has limited control over a wide range of these items. In the following example, both Ps have a total of 36 tokens; the wider lexical range of the first P is summarized in his Type-Token Ratio (36 tokens, 10 types → 0.28), which is more than twice that of the second P (36 tokens, 4 types → 0.11). Such ratios, when used for the lexicon as a whole, provide important indications of lexical range and balance.

Pronominal	
1 me 3 mine 1	Dem that 5 those 2
2 you 4	Art a 4 the 9
3 he 5 him 2 his 1	Other

Pronominal	
1 me 9	Dem that 15
2 you 7	Art
3 him 5	Other

(In calculating item types, contracted forms are conflated with full forms, e.g. *is* and *'s* are considered a single item type.)

5.6.6 The final form of PRISM page 2 is given on p. 149.

Items are assigned to the relevant section of this page, as they occur in data samples. For example, the following sentences occurred in one sample; page 2 items are indicated as appropriate.

I been going about two weeks	Pronominal (1), Verb (*be*), Prepositional (Temp)
Mrs Parker sees me	Proper Name, Pronominal (1)
those are very nice	Pronominal (Dem), Verb (*be*)
and the playground is big	Connective, Pronominal (Art), Verb (*be*)
it's as big as a field	Pronominal (3), Verb (*be*), Other (*as . . . as*), Pronominal (Art)
no	Social (Response)
in a car-park	Prepositional (Loc), Pronominal (Art)
not really	Verb (Neg)
our gerbil did died	Pronominal (1), Verb (Other)
soon I'll be six	Pronominal (1), Verb (Other), Verb (*be*)

5.7 While the items classified in 5.6 are among the most frequently occurring in the language, they do not even begin to account for the range and depth of lexical expression. Indeed, they would be considered marginal items, in any semantic investigation. The bulk of a semantic enquiry is taken up with the analysis of the items which convey most of the information in a sentence—items such as *chair, man, run, garage, big, fat, quickly.* These constitute the majority of a language's lexicon, and provide the most immediate goal of remedial work in semantics. They therefore take up most of the space on the profile chart, their classification in fact covering all of pages 3 to 15.

5.7.1* The following linguistic principle was used, to arrive at this classification. Lexical items are not usually encountered as single items, in isolation

PRISM-L
Minor Lexemes (Summary)

Unanalysed	Unintelligible	Ambiguous	Symbolic Noise	Other		Totals
Social	Spontaneous		Response			
	Stereotype		Comment			
	Proper N		Other			
Relational	Pronominal 1 2 3		Dem Art Other			
	Prepositional Loc		Temp	Other Problems		

	Verbal
	be 1
	  2
	  3
			Other	Neg		

	Interrogative		Tags			
	Connective					
	Empty		Other		Ty	
					To	
Avoidance					Ty	
					To	

from context. It is normal in language learning to be exposed to sets of items relating to a particular theme, such as the weather, music, furniture, fruit or sports. Clinical teaching also aims to work according to this principle, and any semantic profile ought therefore to reflect it. PRISM-L does not therefore begin by listing individual lexical items (e.g. in terms of their frequency, alphabetic order, usefulness), but presents a view of vocabulary as being organized into areas, or *fields*. For example, the field of FRUIT contains such lexical items as *apple, orange, banana,* and *plum.* The assumption is that, as children learn their lexicon, they 'think' of the lexical items as 'belonging' to a semantic field—in other words, that they 'know' that such items as *apple, pear* etc. 'belong together'. The inverted commas around several crucial terms in this sentence reflect our theoretical uncertainty as to what exactly the processes of semantic acquisition are; but the assumption is precise enough to enable a useful model to be constructed for clinical purposes, and this is what PRISM-L attempts to do. The first sections represent fields which are the earliest encountered by a normal child in the course of acquisition; later sections represent his movements into more advanced fields. The acquisitional ordering is, unfortunately, only suggestive, even for the early period. Very little research into the order of acquisition of lexical items has been carried on. The PRISM ordering is based on a synthesis of the findings to date, supplemented by the use of logical criteria, especially for the later stages. What emerges is a lexical classification, a little along the lines of Roget's thesaurus, but operating at a lexical level chosen for its relevance to P's needs in comprehension and production. There is no semantic field 'nautical' separately specified, for example, simply because sailors and sailing are not a common feature of clinical interactions, which tend to concentrate on such topics as home, school, work, relatives, and so on. It is the clinically frequent topics which receive closest attention, therefore; infrequent topics (such as sailing) receive their lexical classification under Other (see further, 5.7.2).

5.7.2 Each page of the profile deals with one or two major themes, summarized as follows:

4	5	6	7	8	9
Human Form and Function		Activity and Sensory		Leisure	Transport

10	11	12	13	14	15
Fauna,	Flora and Elements	Domestic Setting	Dimensions	Institutions and the World	

These notions are too general to provide a classification which would be at all discriminating, but they do help to provide a sense of the organization of the chart as a whole. Rather more useful is the next stage of classification, where a set of 61 major semantic fields is postulated:

4	5	6	7	8	9
Man	Clothing	Moving	Sound	Recreation	Road
		Making/doing	Sight	Occasions	Rail
		Happening	Smell		
Body		Living	Taste	Shows	Air
		Having	Touch	Music	Water
	Food	Thinking	Language		
Health		Feeling	Imagination	Art	Fuel

10	11	12	13	14	15
Animals	Flowers	Building	Quantity	Government	Space
	Trees		Measurement	Law	World
Birds	Light	Furniture	Size	Education	Minerals
	Colour		Shape	Religion	Weapons
Fish	Fire	Tools	Time	Business	Money
			Location		
Insects	Water	Containers	State	Manufacture	Other

But even this level of classification is some way away from the level at which T tends to work. Within each of these major fields, therefore, a set of subfields is postulated, with the aim of breaking down the lexicon into areas that are specific enough to provide a basis for assessment and guidelines for remedial work. It would, of course, be possible to further classify each of these subfields (as with any micro-profile—cf. 1.9.4), but the present level has been found to be sufficiently discriminating for most practical purposes, with 239 subfields being specifically named (there are also several Other categories used). To illustrate this level of lexical organization, each of the major fields is presented below (pp. 152–63), with the various subfields filled in with typical lexemes.

5.7.3* All lexical items, other than those already dealt with on page 2, are assigned to one or other of these semantic fields. Generally, this procedure is straightforward, e.g. *daddy* is Family (p.4), *eyes* are Face (p.4). But there are many cases where it is not possible to be certain about which field a lexical item should be assigned to, or where two or more fields seem equally relevant. For example, *fix* is a specific activity which, in isolation, one would place under Making/Doing on p.6; but in the context of someone saying he was *fixing his car,* one might think it just as reasonable to put the item under Action (re road vehicle) on p.9. Or again, *hospital* might be Health (Other) or Buildings (Type).

Faced with a case of uncertain assignment, the first thing to do is to check that context has been taken fully into account. *Cold,* in the sense of illness, will be placed under Disease (p. 4), whereas in the sense of daily temperature, it will be placed under Climate (p.15). *Toilet,* when it is the

Lexeme Inventory (Major Items)

Man						
Family	sister	relations		Type	youth	grown-up
mother	son			male	lady	baby
grandpa	aunt			female	bachelor	child
wife	cousin			boy	chap	
				girl		
Jobs	painter			General		
farmer	postman			human		
plumber	gardener			person		
milkman				people		
Group	army			Contacts	guest	
crowd	tribe			friend	enemy	
gang	club			neighbour	stranger	
rally	society			schoolfriend		
Location				Other		
Australian	Chinese					
Eskimo						
Scot						
Character +	friendly	—	cowardly	Neutral		
jolly	wise	vain	strange	busy		
eager	noble	unfriendly	dishonest	awake		
interesting	honest	lazy				
		dull				

Body						
Main Parts				Limbs	knee	foot
head	shoulder	back		arm	hand	
neck	chest	bottom		leg	ankle	
limb	waist	tummy		elbow	finger	
Face	ear			Outside		
nose	jaw			skin	beard	
teeth	eye			nail	moustache	
chin	forehead			hair		
Health	disease			Inside	stomach	
clean	catching			skull	lung	
ill	better			bone	nerve	
fever	well			blood	vein	
Character +		—		Neutral		
beautiful	graceful	ugly	awkward	hot		
slender	strong	fat	weak	cool		
handsome		skinny				
Other						

Health						
Disease	infection	ache		Protection	chemist's	
cold	flu	deaf		medicine	clinic	
cough	allergy			pill	hospital	
mumps	polio			prescription	operation	
				ward	therapy	
People	dentist			Implements	needle	thermometer
doctor	patient			drill	splint	stethoscope
surgeon				tooth brush	dressing	bandage
nurse				filling	ointment	plaster
Other						

Clothing							
General	costume	fit		Material	fur		
dress	change	hang up		cotton	cloth		
uniform	put on	take off		nylon	silk		
fashion	wear			fabric	wool		
Outer	cap	jacket		Footwear	sandals		
glove	hood	leggings		boot	socks		
mitten	hat			shoe			
scarf	coat			slippers			
Man	underpants	Woman		Neutral		Child	
tie		bikini	blouse	suit	jeans	nappy	
shirt		gown	skirt	sweater	trousers	rompers	
trunks		dress	nightie	pyjamas			
Accessories	purse			Parts	sleeve	button	
ear-rings	handbag			bow	cuff	hem	
necklace	bracelet			collar	ribbon		
hanky	cufflinks			pocket	zip		
Caring	laundry	tailor	patch	Other			
wash	needle	cobbler	mend				
iron	thread	knit					
dry-clean	washing machine						

Food (Grown)					
Fruit		Part		Location	
apple	grape	pip	stem	bush	orchard
plum	nuts	skin	core	tree	patch
berry		peel		vine	
Vegetables		Grain		Part	
pea	turnip	wheat	corn	stalk	leaf
carrot		rice		root	husk
potatoes		oats		pod	
Character		Other			
sweet	raw				
juicy	rotten				
ripe	delicious				

(Processed)					
Type	pie	sandwich	Dairy		Seafood
jam	cereal		butter	eggs	fish
soup	cake		yoghurt	cheese	shrimp
bread	biscuit		ice-cream		oyster
Drinks			Flavouring		
coffee	pop		salt	sauce	
milk	juice		pepper	vinegar	
tea			sugar		

Food (Grown and processed)						
Action	bake	bite	swallow	Location	butchers	dining room
cook	boil	eat	feed	fridge	grocers	
serve	fry	sip		freezer	restaurant	
preserve	mix	digest		kitchen	cafe	
Meals				Utensils	cup	glass
breakfast	tea			saucepan	knife	bowl
lunch	snack			pot	fork	oven
dinner				kettle	plate	
People	butcher			Other		
waitress	baker					
chef						
cook						

Moving	Come/Go leave wander come arrive appear go get in reach get in return enter follow	Static rest stand lie stay sit lean stop wait
	Sleep wake up doze asleep snore dream	Animate dawdle move sneak run bustle walk hop march
	Things bring drop shut push send bend throw drag take put cut carry lift open melt	Other
Making/ Doing	General finish do try help make attempt use fail start able	Specific arrange smash build mend fix join organise shape
	Type easy simple quickly job boring possible thorough task hard well work difficult easily	Other
Happening	occur pause event reason happen carry on situation cause result end accident start activity luck stop fact chance	Other
Living	live kill life grow become alive breathe birth dead die develop	Other
Having	Process + keep find owner have save discover property own collect accept get gather borrow	Process – miss lose lack waste loss need
Thinking	Process remember believe know understand decide guess forget choose agree think	General thought mystery brain idea puzzle mind plan memory belief
	Type stupid clever silly careful certain crafty	Other
Feeling	+ excited like amuse happy love smile interested hopeful joy enjoy friendly delighted peace laugh	– hate worry glare afraid sad detest cross angry anxious cry jealous bored upset sigh
	Neutral serious proud	Other

Sound	General noise sound pitch	loudness silence hearing listen		Quality quiet noisy low	shrill aloud deafening	
	Specific buzz mutter din	laugh cry moan squeal	bang	Implements hearing-aid loudspeaker microphone		Other
Sight	Act see gaze watch	peer stare glance notice	recognize display have a look view	Implements glasses camera telescope	contacts	Other
Smell	Act sniff smell inhale			Character fragrance perfume stink	spicy musty	Other
Taste	Act taste savour			Character salty sweet sour	bitter tasty delicious	Other
Touch	Act feel handle hold	brush stroke rub pinch	scratch	Character smooth rough soft	cold sticky slimy	wet	Other
Language	Speak/Listen talk shout say	speak whisper listen	rhythm voice	Read/Write read write post deliver	letter alphabet punctuation comma	stamp
	Act argue explain tell	promise order welcome blame	sermon conversation prayer	Product poem poster book	letter magazine card directory	dictionary label
	People printer poet librarian	author postman		Character clear precise vague	boring succinct	
	Implements typewriter pen paper	tape-recorder telephone letterbox dial	Part title cover page picture	word vowel intonation	Other	
Imagination	Type story fairy tale novel	legend adventure pretend	People witch genie fairy	villain hero pixie dwarf	ogre ghost	Other

Recreation	Action	skip		Location	playground
	skate	catch		beach	playroom
	swing	kick		gym	field
	hide	play		park	pitch
	Games	ball		Sports	
	cards	toy		football	
	dominoes			tennis	
	bingo			cricket	
	People	player		Equipment	
	goalie	athlete		ball	
	referee	team		bat	
	linesman	side		goalposts	
	Things	swing	doll	Other	
	kite	slide	plasticine		
	yo-yo	sledge	puzzle		
	marbles	tricycle	game		

Occasions	General		Xmas	Jesus		Other	
	present		tree	shepherds		Easter egg, etc.	
	card		holly				
	gift		carol				

Shows	Type	film	radio	Location	stage	
	play	TV		theatre	ring	
	opera	circus		cinema	arena	
	ballet	parade		fairground		
	Action	juggle		People	actor	
	act			comedian	acrobat	
	perform			dancer	clown	
	dance			musician	audience	
	Implements	mask	trapeze	Other		
	set	wig	costume			
	screen	camera	prize			
	scenery	puppet	roundabouts			

Music	Instruments			Type	tuneful	jazz
	orchestra	band		hymn	catchy	symphony
	trumpet	violin		song	pop	concert
	clarinet			melodic	rock	
	Action			People		
	play			conductor	singer	
	sing			player	drummer	
	listen			composer		
	Parts			Other		
	rhythm	key				
	note					
	beat					

Art	Implements			Type	pottery	
	brush	chisel		drawing	carving	
	pen	paint		picture	trace	
	crayon	chalk		scene		
	Quality		People		Other	
	good	original	artist			
	colourful		painter			
	abstract		sculptor			

Land (Road)	Vehicle	bus	Parts	wheel	
	car	bulldozer	brakes	gears	
	tractor	van	windscreen	handlebars	
	taxi	bike	bumper	pedals	
	Action	skid	Location	hill	signs
	ride	crash	road	curb	
	drive	slow down	street	crossroads	
	steer	collision	pavement	lights	
	People	rider	Other		
	driver	hitch-hiker			
	passenger				
	pedestrian				
(Rail)	Vehicle		Parts		
	train	underground	engine	funnel	
	express		coach	bumpers	
	freight		guards van		
	Action		Location		
	drive		rails	level crossing	
	shunt		station	track	
			platform		
	People		Other		
	guard	ticket inspector			
	driver				
	passenger				
Air	Vehicle	balloon	Parts	propellor	
	plane	helicopter	tail	cockpit	
	jet		wing	seat	
	glider		rotor		
	Action	dive	Location		
	fly	glide	airport	control tower	
	take off	parachute	runway		
	land		hangar		
	People		Other		
	pilot	crew			
	stewardess	passenger			
Water	Vehicle	submarine	Parts		
	boat	tanker	rudder	bow	
	ship	yacht	helm	propellor	
	navy	dinghy	deck		
	Action		Location		
	row	float	port	dock	
	sail	sink	harbour		
	steam		pier		
	People		Other		
	seaman	crew			
	sailor				
	captain				
Fuel	gas	antifreeze	power	Other	
	oil	paper	steam		
	diesel	wood			
	coal	electricity			

Animals	General creature beast mammal			Pet horse　gerbil dog　rabbit kitten		
	Farm horse　pig sheep　goat cow　donkey			Wild(Small) fox　rabbit otter　mouse mole　squirrel		
	Water octopus　frog whale　newt seal　crab			Wild (Large) bear　tiger　monkey lion　panda　elephant wolf　reindeer		
	Reptile crocodile　lizard snake　slug worm			Extinct/Imaginary dinosaur　dodo dragon　diplodocus unicorn		
	Noise　bleat bark　snarl meow　roar neigh			Location zoo　hutch cage　jungle kennel　burrow		
	Action (Us → Them) trap　catch　herd shear　ride　shoot breed　snare			(Them → Us) bite　hibernate kill　pounce spit　trot		
	Type tame　vicious gentle　intelligent obedient		Parts hoof　head leg　mane rib	Other		
Birds	Type　ostrich　owl robin　parrot　emu thrush　budgie lark　pheasant			Parts feather　beak claw　wing tail　crest		
	Water swan　puffin duck　gull penguin　heron			Farm chicken　turkey duck goose		
	Action fly　roost　moult migrate　lay　sing dive　perch			Noise chirp　quack screech　caw call　cluck		Other
Fish	Type cod　goldfish salmon　pike shark　eel			Parts gill fin scales		
	Action swim　catch dive spawn			Control trawler　hook net　rod bait　fisherman		Other
Insects	Type　fly　spider ant　wasp　grasshopper beetle　bee flea　butterfly			Parts feelers　antennae thorax　wing leg		
	Action　sting crawl　swarm bite　buzz		Location hive nest	Other		

Flowers (etc.)	Type	bouquet	fragrant		Parts	petal	
	rose	bed			root	seed	
	tulip	lily			stem		
	daisy	brilliant			bud		
	Action	bloom	arrange		Other		
	grow	blossom	prune				
	bud	pick					
	die	plant					
Trees	Type	oak			Parts	stump	
	apple	gnarled			bud	trunk	
	birch	tall			bark	branch	
	pine	shady			root	bough	
	Action	prune			Other		
	grow						
	fell						
	chop						
Light	Type	flash	flickering		Control		Other
	dark	glow	dim		candle	lighthouse	
	Light	shine	bright		lamp		
	shade	glare	dazzling		bulb		
Colour	Type	deep			General		
	red	warm			hue		
	orange	pale			shade		
	vivid	gaudy			tint		
	Action	brush			Implement		Other
	paint	spray			brush	ink	
	dye				crayon		
	stain				paint		
Fire	Type	smoke	ashes		Fuel	paper	
	fire	scorch	hot		oil	wood	
	spark	burn			gas		
	flame	smoulder			coal		
	Control	hose			Other		
	extinguisher	brigade					
	matches	stove					
	fireman	fireplace					
Water	Type	cold	tide		Action	trickle	condense
	wet	lukewarm			boil	drip	pour
	shallow	rushing			flood	sprinkle	pump
	clear	wave			flow	splash	
	Control	sink			Other		
	canal	pipe					
	drain	fountain					
	tap	reservoir					

Building	Type	castle	flat	Parts	roof	rooms
	house	igloo	home	window	door	stairs
	bungalow	hotel		ceiling	floor	hall
	cottage	tent		wall	balcony	
	Outside	gate		Materials		
	garage	lawn		glass	plaster	
	garden	car park		tile	cement	
	drive	doormat		brick		
	Action	repair	mop	People		
	clean	build	duster	architect	electrician	
	sweep	mend		bricklayer	painter	
	polish	mow		maid	handyman	
	Rooms	kitchen		Other		
	playroom	basement				
	cellar	study				
	bathroom					
Furniture	General	cupboard	table	Bathroom		
	chair	curtain	telephone	toilet	shower	
	shelf	mirror	picture	tap		
	carpet	lamp		bath		
	Bedroom			Living Room		
	bed	mattress		sofa	TV	
	wardrobe			armchair	hi-fi	
	dressing-table			piano		
	Kitchen/Dining			Other		
	sink	stove				
	sideboard					
	fridge					
Tools	General	shovel	screw	Farm/Garden		
	hammer	cut	ladder	hoe	shears	mow
	drill	nails	kit	rake	spade	weed
	saw	hinge	bench	mower	barrow	axe
	People			Other		
	painter					
	plumber					
	gardener					
Containers	Type	safe	jug	bag	Parts	door
	basket	handbag	can	bowl	top	side
	parcel	case	bottle		lid	lock
	purse	cupboard	box		handle	
	Action	fill		Other		
	open	pack				
	close	empty				
	lock	bulging				

Quantity	General only even enough several odd every else bit lot(s) all		Specific one half alone two single dozen pair trio	
	Act add count divide		Other	

Measurement	Distance inch mile foot ruler cm	Weight ounce gram scales	Volume pint litre barrel
	Time second century hour calendar season clock	Heat degree Fahrenheit thermometer	Other

Size	+ deep high heavy big great long expand large huge thick widen tall giant wide	– thin narrow shrink small narrow reduce tiny short lower little light

Shape	line square round stripe bump dot block bent pile corner circle ball flat spot hole pyramid crooked pointed heap		

Time	Day dawn evening morning midnight noon		Period instant ancient age youth lifetime young term old	
	Past yesterday just recently ago previous	Present now today	Future soon tomorrow next	
	Frequency never again always once daily often sometimes		Other	

Location	General here further position there absent spot everywhere far distance		Specific left outside north upstairs address south forwards right indoors	
	Part centre top bottom summit middle side		Other	

State	Quality best good nice better awful		Intensity actually very really at all just	
	Like + equal group alike matching compare same twin sort out similar series also		Like – different other opposite contrast unlike	
	Other			

Government	Type			People		Other
	country	town		civil servant		vote
	council	county	capital	cabinet minister		election
	parliament	city		king		
	national	borough		mayor		

Law	Location	People	Other
	prison	lawyer criminal	arrest
	court	police	trial
	police station	judge	

Education	Type		Part	
	school nursery		classroom cloakroom	
	university		playground desk	
	college		blackboard	
	Action		People	
	study teach		teacher student	
	learn		pupil lecturer	
	instruct		head secretary	
	Topic		Other	
	history			
	English			
	number work			

Religion	Location		Implements	
	church shrine		candle altar	
	cathedral		pulpit cross	
	temple		bible organ	
	People		Other	
	priest nun			
	rabbi sister			
	vicar			

Business	Type		Implements		
	banking advertising		files computer		
	insurance		typewriter		
	publishing		duplicator		
	Action buy		People secretary barber		
	type organise		manager owner florist		
	sell display		salesman cashier		
	advertise		customer grocer		
	Location office block		Parts	Other	
	supermarket toyshop		sign counter		
	boutique hairdressers		lift shelf		
	department store		escalator		

Manufacturing	Location		Equipment		
	factory workshop		machine(ry) conveyor		
	mill		lathe computer		
	laboratory		tools		
	Action		People	Other	
	make operate		worker engineer		
	produce sell		manager technician		
	design		foreman		

Space	Entities/Events sun eclipse moon orbit planet		Exploration rocket astronaut capsule observatory lift-off	Other
World	Land jungle beach continent woods mountain meadow valley coast		Water river sea pond channel stream lake	
	Surface rock ground ice soil snow sand		Depth cave well underground tunnel	
	Location map pole globe abroad equator	Climate cloud icy humid hot rain drizzle storm weather fog frost thunder temperature sunny		Other
Minerals	Type gold copper metal oil coal	Act bore prospect mine dynamite blast pump		Other
Weapons	Type gun spear rifle missile bomb stone		People hunter enemy trapper army	Other
Money	Units penny cheque pound dollar 5p		Location bank purse wallet safe	
	Action sell save invest spend waste buy advertise	Type wages cheap tax expensive cost savings		Other
Other				

name of a whole room, will be placed under Parts (of building) (p.12); but when it refers to the specific object within a room, it will be placed under Furniture (presumably Bathroom, in most cases) (also p.12).

However, even after taking context into account, there will still be some unclear cases. This is in the nature of semantic field modelling: the real world does not present itself as a set of neat compartments, to which lexical items may be assigned. Just because some fields are reasonably clear (such as colour, body-parts, containers), it does not follow that all fields will be so easy to define; and some overlapping is inevitable. It is part of the meaning of *hospital,* for instance, to involve Health *and* Building. The consequences of this must therefore be anticipated, if a consistent procedure is to be introduced. The solution adopted is an arbitrary one, but it is preferred over the alternative (which some theoreticians have suggested), namely to jettison the semantic fields notion altogether. In cases where T is uncertain as to whether a lexeme should be assigned to field A or field B, it is assigned to *both* fields, with the less certain assignment indicated by the use of square brackets. For example, *fix* above could be assigned to both Making/Doing and Action (Road vehicle), and T would mark one or other of these with square brackets. If he cannot decide which of the two assignments to mark with square brackets, the convention is to leave the earliest item in the procedure unmarked: in the present example, if there were uncertainty between Making/Doing and Action (of Road vehicle), the Making/Doing assignment would be left unmarked, as it occurs on p.6, whereas the other assignment is later in the procedure, on p.9. Such a convention is needed, in order to ensure that items do not get counted twice, when arriving at totals in P's vocabulary—only unbracketed items are included in the totalling-up procedure.

5.7.4 To illustrate the field-assignment procedure in more detail, the remaining lexemes used in the sentences in 5.6.6 would be processed as follows:

Item	Lexeme	Major Field	Subfield	Page
going	GO	Moving	Come/Go	6
two	TWO	Quantity	Specific	13
weeks	WEEK	Measurement	Time	13
sees	SEE	Sight	Act	7
very	VERY	State	Intensity	13
nice	NICE	State	Quality	13
playground	PLAYGROUND	Recreation	Location	8
big	BIG	Size	+	13
field	FIELD	World	Land	14
car-park	CAR-PARK	Land(Road)	Location	9
really	REALLY	State	Intensity	13
gerbil	GERBIL	Animal	Pet	10
died	DIE	Living	—	6
soon	SOON	Time	Future	13
six	SIX	Measurement	Time	13

The relatively abstract nature of this P's vocabulary can be seen from the frequent use of p.13. By contrast, the following section of items shows a much less mature lexicon (taken from a sample of free conversation, using farm animals as stimulus, with a severely-delayed child of 4):

Item	Lexeme	Major Field	Subfield	Page
pig	PIG	Animals	Farm	10
cow	COW	Animals	Farm	10
mummy (cow)	MUMMY	Animals	Other	10
gone	GO	Moving	Come/Go	6
mans	MAN	Man	Type	4
eat	EAT	Food	Action	5
sleeping	SLEEP	Moving	Sleep	6
look	LOOK	Sight	Act	7
tractor	TRACTOR	Land(Road)	Vehicle	9
horsie	HORSE	Animals	Farm	10
quack-quack	QUACK	Animals	Noise	10
there	THERE	Location	General	13

5.7.5 It will be evident, from the repeated use of certain fields in each of these examples, that a single short sample will not suffice to provide a representative picture of P's lexicon. Normal conversation proceeds thematically, with certain topics being introduced and explored, before new topics are moved on to. The more reluctant the P, and the more structured the situation, the fewer topics will be covered. To obtain a general sense of P's lexical range, therefore, a series of samples will have to be taken, and a cumulative analysis made; and this has consequences for the way in which items are marked on the chart and totalled. It is necessary to introduce a convention so that the lexemes used in one sample are not confused with those used in another. There are many possible ways of keeping samples apart, using different colours, symbols, etc. One of the most convenient procedures is simply to assign each sample a number (see further, 5.7.9) and use this to separate groups of occurrences, in the following way:

man 1 卅| 2 |||| 4 卅

would mean that in sample 1, P used *man* 6 times; in sample 2 he used it a further 4 times; in sample 3 not at all (so not mentioned); and in sample 4 a further 5 times.

5.7.6 Page 3 of the chart is used as a summary of the numbers of items used in the various major fields. In the upper part of each box, the total number of lexeme *types* for a particular field is given; in the lower part, the total number of lexeme *tokens*. If different samples are taken, the totals are written in from left to right. For example:

MAN	**1**	7	**2**	4	**3**	16
		24		11		29

would mean that in the first sample, P used 24 lexeme tokens from the field Man, but only 7 lexeme types; in the second, there were 11 tokens, but only 4 types; and in the third, there were 29 tokens from 16 types. If one wished, an average for the whole series could be obtained (namely, 64 tokens for 27 types, a ratio of 0.42); but on the whole, statistics relating to individual fields do not turn out to be so useful as a single statistic relating to P's use of *all* major lexemes. The totals at the top of p.3 thus relate to the page as a whole.

We can see this procedure in operation if we take the summary page from a PRISM chart of the 4-year-old child referred to above (see p. 167). In P's first sample, 101 lexeme tokens represented 37 lexeme types (a TTR of 0.38); in the second sample, 97 tokens represented 50 types (TTR of 0.52). P's vocabulary is evidently far less repetitive in the second sample, though some lexemes are still being frequently used (in Animals and Location, in particular). One would need to look back at the individual fields to assess the significance of these totals, of course: in the present example, the frequent use of the lexeme *pig* was explained by the way P was playing; on the other hand, the frequent use of the lexeme *there* (under Location) was interpreted as a sign of weakness, it being used by P where more advanced children would have introduced specific nouns.

5.7.7* The final page of PRISM-L (see p. 168) provides space for T to note items which provide evidence of P's emerging semantic system—that is, of the way in which P is relating lexemes. Three types of relationship are recognized.

(a) Paradigmatic relations include the relationships of sense often referred to as *synonymy, opposition, hyponymy* and *incompatibility*. For example, if P were to say, about a cup, *it's broken/ – smashed/*, the fact that he is using these two lexemes synonymously would be noted on p.16 (they would also have been logged under their appropriate semantic field (Happening)). If he were to say, *that's not dirty/ it's clean/*, the use of these lexemes as opposites would be noted on p.16. Likewise, for *a rose is a sort of flower,* where the relationship between *rose* and *flower* is one of hyponymy (or class-inclusion); and for *that's not blue/ it's green/*, where *blue* and *green* are incompatible terms from the same lexical system (Colour). In each case, the items in question would be noted on p.16, in addition to their placement under individual semantic fields. Some clinical tasks, of course, concentrate on these points ('What's another word for . . . ?', 'What's the opposite of . . . ?', and so on); their emergence in P's free conversation, at an early stage in semantic development, is an important indication of progress.

(b) Syntagmatic relations refer to the way in which lexemes go together in expected sequences, as when *letters* are *posted* in *pillar-boxes,* or one *cooks food* in a *pan.* Some lexeme-sequences are so fixed that they are said to be idiomatic (e.g. *raining cats and dogs*). On p.16, one notes any idiomatic phrases which would not be easily located under individual semantic fields, along with any evidence of P's developing awareness of lexical cooccurrences. For example, *kick ball, drink tea, post letter.* Not every sequence will be noted, but only those where there is a particularly close relationship between the lexemes. There would be no point in noting such sequences as *see + house, go + road* or *have + toy,* for example.

Major Lexemes (Summary)

Totals Ty	37	.38	50	.52	
To	101		97		

Page						
4	Man		Body		Health	
	¹6 ²7		¹1 ²4			
	11 9		1 6			
5	Clothing		Food			
	¹1		¹3 ²6			
	1		9 10			
6	Moving		Making/Doing		Happening	Living
	¹4 ²7		²3			
	15 11		8			
	Having		Thinking		Feeling	
			²1		¹1	
			1		1	
7	Sound	Sight		Smell	Taste	Touch
		²2				
		2				
	Language		Imagination			
	¹1					
	2					
8	Recreation	Occasions		Shows	Music	Art
	¹1					
	1					
9	Road	Rail		Air	Water	Fuel
	¹2 ²4					
	4 7					
10	Animals	Birds		Fish		Insects
	¹3 ²4	²1				
	14 11	1				
11	Flowers		Trees		Light	
			²2			
			2			
	Colour		Fire		Water	
	²1				¹1	
	1				1	
12	Building		Furniture		Tools	Containers
	¹3 ²4		¹4			
	10 7		11			
13	Quantity	Measurement		Size		Shape
	¹1 ²2			¹1		
	5 7			4		
	Time		Location		State	
	¹1		¹1 ²2			
	1		9 14			
14	Government	Law	Education	Religion	Business	Manufacture
15	Space	World		Minerals	Weapons	Money
	¹1					
	1					
	Other					

Further Analysis

Paradigmatic Relations	Synonymy	Error
	Opposition	
	Hyponymy	
	Incompatibility	
	Other	
Syntagmatic Relations		
Developmental Error	Overextension	
	Underextension	
	Mismatch	

The point of having these sections is often clearer when one sees the errors which Ps make in the use of syntagmatic or paradigmatic relations, and any errors are noted in a separate column on the right of p.16. For example, *I eat my milk* would be logged as a syntagmatic error on p.16 (in addition to assigning *eat* and *milk* to the appropriate sections of the Food field). *That not big/ – it pretty/* would be logged as a paradigmatic error (of opposition), insofar as it seemed that P was using *big* as the opposite of *pretty* (again, both items would have been assigned to their appropriate semantic fields earlier in the chart).

(c) Lastly, under Developmental Error are placed any lexemes where there is evidence that P has an immature understanding of the meaning involved. Three categories are generally recognized under this heading:

the lexeme is *overextended* in production, e.g. *dog* being used for all animals;
the lexeme is *underextended* in production, e.g. *dog* being used for the family dog only, and not for other kinds of dog;
there is a *mismatch* between P's use and normal adult use, i.e. no obvious point of contact between them, e.g. a *window* referred to as a *happy*.

Analogous errors in adult P use would also be classified under these headings.

It should be appreciated that it is often not possible to be certain as to P's overextension, underextension or mismatch, in a spontaneous speech sample. For the few instances where such problems are in evidence, there are likely to be many others where the evidence is ambiguous or unobtainable. The instances noted in this section of the chart, therefore, can only ever be illustrative of a trend.

5.7.8 There is one other factor which it is helpful to bear in mind when interpreting lexical use—whether the item is a *repetition* of an item in T's stimulus sentence, or a self-repetition. Repetition is here defined as it is for the LARSP procedure (though without the criterion of prosodic identity): to count as a repetition, an item in P's sentence must be the same lexeme as one which occurred in T's *immediately* preceding sentence, or be a repetition by P of an item he has used in his *immediately* preceding sentence. For example, in the following extract, the repeated items are italicized:

T	is he in a car/	
P	*car/*	*repetition (T)*
	yes/	
	a car/	
T	and where's the car going/	
P	*car* shops/	*repetition (T)*
	shops/	*repetition (self)*
	go to *shops/*	*repetition (T)*
T	what's he going to buy in the shops/	*repetition (self)*
P	don't know/	
T	will he buy some bread/ –	
	has he got enough money/ do you think/	
P	buy bread/	
	buy bread/	*repetition (self) (twice)*

The notion of repetition is useful only for the analysis of major lexemes (i.e. excluding those logged on page 2). Repeated items are indicated on the chart by dots instead of ticks (though any other graphic convention would do as well); for example *man* |···||··|· would mean that this lexeme was used spontaneously 4 times and was repeated 6 times. The repetitions total is given on page 1 of the procedure.

5.7.9 Page 1 of the PRISM-L procedure (see p. 171) is a summary of the samples used and the main statistical findings. Each sample is given a line, with successive samples numbered in sequence. The date, duration and type of sample is given. Then, for each sample, the following totals are added:

total Unanalysed items (from the top of p.2);
total Minor types (the sum of Social, Relational and Avoidance, on p.2);
total Minor tokens (the sum of Social, Relational and Avoidance, on p.2);
type-token ratio for Minor items (i.e. total types divided by total tokens);
total Major types (from all the semantic fields);
total Major tokens (from all the semantic fields—including repetitions);
type-token ratio for Major items;
the ratio of Minor tokens to Major tokens (total Minor divided by total Major);
the number of semantic fields represented in the sample;
the number of subfields represented in the sample (including Others);
total Repetitions of Major items.

A space is provided for any general comments T may wish to add.

The illustration below is of two samples from the same child. The Minor column shows frequent use of a few minor items, and a consequent low TTR, for both samples. The Major column shows an increase in the number of lexeme types and tokens from one sample to the next (though their proportions stay approximately the same). This increase was achieved despite the fact that fewer fields and subfields were in use during the second sample. There were also fewer repetitions, in the second sample. The proportion of minor to major tokens has also improved, and is close to the ratio one would expect in normal samples.

5.8 Lexical items do not occur in isolation from grammar: they are a part of a sentence sequence, whether T's or P's, which itself has a semantic function to perform. Each sentence, in fact, can be viewed from a semantic as well as a grammatical point of view. Instead of referring to *the cat bit the dog* as a 'Subject-Verb-Object' construction (cf. 2.11.1), we could refer to it as an 'Actor-Action-Goal' construction—in other words, identifying the *functions,* or *roles,* that the grammatical units perform in the communication of meaning. A lexical item may have quite different roles, depending on where it is used in a sentence: compare, for example, *the cat bit the dog,* where the cat is 'Actor', and *the dog bit the cat,* where the cat is 'Goal' or 'Recipient' of the action. Note also that an item may retain its role, even if the grammar changes, as when *the cat bit the dog* becomes *the dog was bitten by the cat*—the cat is 'Actor' in both sentences.

It is therefore important to know, in clinical work, what role P is attributing

PRISM–L
Summary
Name   Joanna H.   Age   3 ; 6   Date of birth   20·8·77

Sample no.	1	2					
Date	2·2·81	24·2·81					
Duration	15 mins.	15 mins.					
Type	Free conversation with T, playing with dolls house and furniture	as previous, but with farm set					
Unanalysed	17	11					
Minor (p2) Types	33	28					
Tokens	189	142					
TTR	·18	·19					
Minor:major (Tokens)	1·52	1·0					
Major (pp4-5) Types	70	81					
Tokens	124	141					
TTR	·56	·57					
Fields used	20	18					
Sub-fields used	39	31					
Repetitions	8	6					

Comments

to a lexical item. When P encounters a lexical item, it is always in a certain sentence role; and when he uses it himself, he must use it in a particular sentence role. If P has difficulties with a lexical item in a certain role, accordingly, this point needs to be made clear on any profile chart. Similarly, if T wants to check that P is able to use a lexical item in all its possible sentence roles, the profile chart should be such that it provides guidelines to this end. It is this concern which motivates the PRISM-G procedure (cf. 5.2). It would have been nice to have incorporated the grammatical information directly onto the PRISM-L chart, but there were too many descriptive dimensions for any practicable design to emerge. The charts are therefore separate, but complementary.

5.9 Five Stages of development are recognized on the PRISM-G chart— though in the absence of empirical research they cannot be clearly related to ages. Stages I–IV deal with the emerging semantic structure of the clause; Stage V deals with clause sequences. In addition, there are sections to handle unanalysed clauses, quantitative summaries, and certain other features of semantic concern. The layout of the three pages is shown below (for details, see pp. 174–5).

Unanalysed	Stage III	Stage V
Stage I		
Stage II	Stage IV	Other
	Totals I–IV	

5.9.1 The Unanalysed section contains the usual range of problems which makes a sentence or clause impossible to analyse (cf. the use of these categories on the LARSP chart, 2.5). Sentences which are *unintelligible,* formally *incomplete* (as marked by prosody or lack of punctuation), containing *symbolic noise,* semantically *ambiguous* or *stereotyped* are given no further analysis. (The absence of a semantically *deviant* category (cf. 2.5.1) from this section is not theoretically motivated, but is simply a consequence of the lack of information about developmental semantic norms (see further, 5.9.11).)

5.9.2* An important theoretical distinction is introduced to handle the data of Stages I to IV. A clause is seen as a sequence of semantic *elements,* corresponding to the clause elements recognized in the grammatical analysis in Chapter 2. These elements, minimally, consist of a single word, as in *John kicked Jim,* where the Subject-Verb-Object sequence can be interpreted semantically as Actor-Activity-Goal (see further below). When these elements consist of more than one word, the semantically most important item is seen as being *specified* in various ways, and the specifications are classified separately. For example, in the sentence *the dog bit two cats in the garden,* there are four elements (Actor-Activity-Goal-Location), and three of these elements are specified, as follows:

dog   specified by   *the*
cats   specified by   *two*
garden   specified by   *in, the*

The set of elements which it is possible to recognize varies somewhat throughout the developmental period: in the earliest Stage, it is very difficult to be precise as to the semantic function of clause elements, and theorists are by no means agreed as to the kind and number of functions it proves useful to work with at later periods of development. For present purposes, only the most important functions are recognized, with less important or unclear functions being assigned to the category of Other. The basic set of functions recognized in the PRISM-G procedure is as follows:

Actor   the animate being that causes an action or change of state, e.g. **John** *kicked the ball, the ball was kicked by* **John.**
Experiencer   the animate being that experiences an action or change of state, e.g. **John** *is happy,* **John** *saw a car.*
Dynamic   an observable activity or change of state, e.g. *kick, go, run.*
Static   a process where there is no observable activity or change of state, e.g. *think, see, know.*
Goal   the object or being which undergoes the result of an action or change of state, e.g. *John kicked* **the ball,** *John saw* **Jim.**
Locative   the location of the action or state specified by the verb, e.g. *he went* **into the garden,** *he is* **there.**
Temporal   the time of the action or state specified by the verb, as expressed outside of the verb phrase, e.g. *we went* **at 7 o'clock,** *he came in* **later.**

Certain additional functions are recognized at Stages I and II, because of their developmental significance; but apart from these, all other functions are grouped under Other (e.g. so-called *instrumental, benefactive, comitative*).
The basic set of specifications used in the PRISM-G procedure is as follows:

Scope   any item (usually a preposition) specifying a locative, temporal manner, purpose, or other such relationship, e.g. **in** *box,* **for** *a car,* **at** *7 o'clock.*
Attribute   any item (usually adjectives, or nouns used adjectivally) which specifies a characteristic or property, e.g. *a* **red** *box, that's* **small,** *a tin of* **Coke.**
Definiteness   the use of definite/indefinite article or the demonstratives, e.g. *in* **a** *box,* **that** *car.*
Possessive   the use of any item specifying possession, e.g. **my** *car,* **John's** *car.*
Quantity   any item (usually a determiner or quantifier) which specifies amount, number etc., e.g. **two** *dogs,* **all** *the bread,* **some** *bread.*

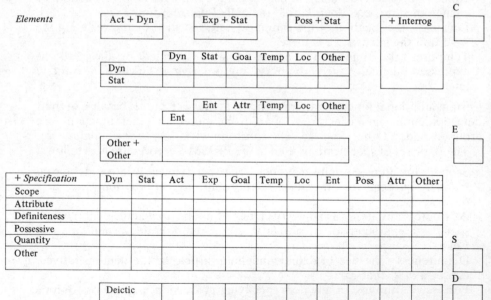

PRISM–G Name ___ Age ___ Sample ___ Totals

Unanalysed
Unintelligible ___ Incomplete ___ Symbolic Noise ___ Ambiguous ___ Stereotypes ___ ☐

I

Minor

Social	Proper Name	Other		+ Specifications

☐

Major C/E ☐

Elements	Activity		Entity		Deictic				Attr	Inter-rog	Other
	Dyn	Stat	Anim	Inanim	Anim	Inanim	Sco	Other	Attr		
Cop											

D ☐

+ Specification											
Scope											
Attribute											
Definiteness											
Possessive											
Quantity											
Other											

S ☐

II C ☐

Elements	Act + Dyn	Exp + Stat	Poss + Stat	+ Interrog

	Dyn	Stat	Goal	Temp	Loc	Other
Dyn						
Stat						

	Ent	Attr	Temp	Loc	Other
Ent					

Other + Other	

E ☐

+ Specification	Dyn	Stat	Act	Exp	Goal	Temp	Loc	Ent	Poss	Attr	Other
Scope											
Attribute											
Definiteness											
Possessive											
Quantity											
Other											

S ☐

Deictic											

D ☐

III

Elements	+ Goal	+ Temp	+ Loc	+ Other		+ Interrog
Act + Dyn						
Exp + Stat						
Poss + Stat						
Dyn + Goal						
Stat + Goal						
Other						

C □

E □

+ Specification	Dyn	Stat	Act	Exp	Poss	Goal	Temp	Loc	Other
Scope									
Attribute									
Definiteness									
Possessive									
Quantity									
Other									
	Deictic								

S □

D □

IV

Elements	+ Temp	+ Loc	+ Other		+ Interrog
Act + Dyn + Goal					
Exp + Stat + Goal					
Poss + Stat + Goal					
Other					

C □

E □

+ Specification	Dyn	Stat	Act	Exp	Poss	Goal	Temp	Loc	Other
Scope									
Attribute									
Definiteness									
Possessive									
Quantity									
Other									
	Deictic								

S □

D □

5+ Elements	
Deictic	+ Specification

C □ E □

D □ S □

Totals		Means	
Major clauses (C)		Elements per clause (E/C)	
Major elements (E)		Specifications per element (S/E)	
Specifications (S)		Deictics per element (D/E)	
Deictics (D)			

Further, or unclear specifications are grouped under the heading of *Other* (e.g. phrasal *and,* as in *and me, boy and girl;* negative particles, as in *he can't;* auxiliary verbs, as in *may go*).

We may now use these notions of element function and element specification as part of the descriptive framework for Stages I to IV.

5.9.3 At Stage I, sentences contain one semantic element only. A distinction is drawn between Minor and Major types of sentence, as on the LARSP chart (2.7), but construed in semantic terms. Minor sentences are semantically unproductive (cf. 5.5): they are divided into Social (e.g. *yes, no, thanks, sorry, please*), proper names (e.g. *John, Mummy, London*) and Others (comment clauses, tags, etc.—cf. 5.6.2 and 5.6.3). Specifications at this stage are uncommon, and are not subclassified: each instance is logged once, as it occurs, in the + Specifications box in the upper right of Stage I, e.g. *to London, very sorry.*

5.9.4* At Stage I, sentences are too short, and context usually too unclear, for a full analysis in terms of semantic functions to be made. The following categories are therefore recognized:

Activity   subclassified into Dynamic and Static, as above.

Entity   subclassified into Animate and Inanimate; for example, sentences such as *màn/, còw/, bòy/* would be analysed as Animate Entity, and *bàll/, càr/, gàrage/* would be Inanimate Entity. It is not possible to be consistent, at this Stage, in assigning such functions as Actor, Goal, Location to these entities—hence the use of the less specific classification.

Deictic items are those which refer directly to spatial or temporal characteristics of the situation in which an utterance takes place (e.g. *there, that, him*). They have a particularly important role to play in normal language acquisition, and their significance in clinical settings has also been noted—deictic items often being used as a means of 'avoiding' more specific lexemes. P's reliance on deictic expression is therefore noted throughout Stages I to IV, and at Stage I, where it is especially common, a more detailed classification of the phenomenon is provided. Four subcategories are recognized: Animate items, such as *him, she, I;* items referring to Inanimate Objects, such as *it, that;* items referring to spatio-temporal Scope, such as *then, there, now, down, top;* and Other possibilities (including cases where the deixis has unclear reference, as when *one* might refer to an animate or an inanimate entity). Numerals without nominal support are also considered to be Deictic (Other), e.g. *T what's hàppened to the 'car/ P twò/* .

Attribute is used in the same sense as above (5.9.2), but whereas in the earlier use the attribute was a specification of some other item, in its present use, it is the *only* item in the sentence, e.g. *T 'look at that càr/ P bìg/.*

Interrogative items are question-words, such as *how, where, who, what for.* When they occur as the only element in a sentence, they are counted under Interr at Stage I. (Interrogatives at later stages are discussed below.)

Other items at this stage may be encountered, e.g. *no* or *not* when used other than as a social minor.

Specification categories are used as in 5.9.2, e.g.

Sentence	Element	Specification
my car	Inanimate Entity	Possessive
a man	Animate Entity	Definiteness
in there	Deictic Scope	Scope
nice car	Inanimate Entity	Attribute
two big cars	Inanimate Entity	Quantity Attribute
all the people	Animate Entity	Quantity Definiteness
very nice	Attribute	Other
where to	Interrogative	Scope
for brushing	Dynamic	Scope
is running	Dynamic	Other
and man	Animate Entity	Other

The procedure is to mark specifications in the same column as that used for marking the element. For example, to mark *my car*, one first locates *car* (in the Inanimate Entity column); *my* is then located along the Possessive line, further down the same column:

Elements	Activity		Entity	
	Dyn	Stat	Anim	Inanim
				I
		Cop		

+ *Specification*				
Scope				
Attribute				
Definiteness				
Possessive				I
Quantity				
Other				

The only other item to note at Stage I is the use of the Copula along with one of the elements Entity, Deictic, Attribute, Interrogative or Other. From a semantic point of view, there is no difference between the meaning of *nice* and *is nice*. It thus seems reasonable to consider both of these as single-element sentences, and to note the copula where it occurs. Thus, *is nice* would be marked as Attribute, with an additional mark on the Copula line, further down the same column:

The same procedure would be used for such other examples as *be there* (Deictic Scope + Copula), *where is* (Interrogative + Copula), *am a boy* (Animate Entity + Copula + Definiteness). (For a similar treatment of the copula at later Stages, see 5.9.4.)

In the Totals column, the following information is recorded:

total Minor sentences, in the box to the right of the Minor section;
total Major sentences, in the box marked C/E (standing for 'clause'/'element', for reasons explained in 5.9.7);
total Deictic items, in the box marked D;
total Specifications, in the box marked S.

The whole of the Stage I procedure may be seen in the following illustration, where a short piece of dialogue is analysed, transferred onto the profile chart, and totalled.

		Element	Specification
T	'show me the shèep/		
P	thère/	Deictic Scope	–
T	that's ríght/		
	and 'where's he gòing/		
P	in thère/	Deictic Scope	Scope
T	in whère/ Míchael/		
P	in field/	Inanimate Entity	Scope
T	'that's rìght/		
	he's 'gone into the field/		
P	and twò shéeps/	Animate Entity	Quantity
	lòok/	Static Activity	Other (*and*)
	gòne/	Dynamic Activity	
T	yês/		
	they've gòne/ hàven't they/		
P	yès/	Social Minor	
	thàt one/ (referring to *sheep*)	Deictic Animate	Definiteness

I

Minor

	Social	Proper Name	Other		+ Specifications	
I						I

Major

Elements	Activity		Entity		Deictic				Attr	Inter-rog	Other	C/E
	Dyn	Stat	Anim	Inanim	Anim	Inanim	Sco	Other				7
	I	I	I	I	I		II					
												D
												3
	Cop											
+ Specification												
Scope				I			I					
Attribute												
Definiteness				I								
Possessive												S
Quantity			I									
Other			I									5

5.9.4* Stage II sentences consist of two major semantic elements, classified according to the functions listed in 5.9.2, insofar as a clear interpretation can be arrived at. The various combinations are listed regardless of the order in which they occur in the clause, e.g. Actor + Dynamic is used for both *man kick* and *kick man* (when the latter means also 'man is kicking'). Examples of the 2-element combinations are as follows:

> Act + Dyn *man go, the man is going, been stung by a wasp*
>   Dyn   Act
> Exp + Stat *man see, I remember, the dog wants to*

Possessor (Poss) is introduced at this point, to handle the frequent use in normal development of the relationship illustrated by *mummy have* (something) or *I got* (something), and other such verbs of possession. Such combinations would be analysed as Poss + Stat.

In the next section, a Dynamic verb or a Static verb is used along with one of the following elements: Dynamic, Static, Goal, Temporal, Locative or Other.

Dyn + Dyn *go kick, come to play*	Stat + Dyn *want to jump, try catch*
Dyn + Stat *go see, open look*	Stat + Stat *want see, try to remember*
Dyn + Goal *kick ball, push a car*	Stat + Goal *see a man, want ice-cream*
Dyn + Temp *kick now, go in minute*	Stat + Temp *see soon, want tomorrow*
Dyn + Loc *go there, push on floor*	Stat + Loc *see in garden, want in there*
Dyn + Other *go not, push nice*	Stat + Other *see lovely, want yes*

In all cases except Dyn + Stat (which also occurs as Stat + Dyn), order is not significant, e.g. both *kick now* and *now kick* are logged as Dyn + Temp.

At this stage of development, there are many clauses where it is not clear what particular function to assign to an item; all that can be said is that some entity has been referred to. In the clause *man there*, for example, the entity *man* is given a location, but it is not possible to say whether *man* is actor (?'man goes there'), experiencer (?'man sees something there'), goal (?'someone has done something to the man there'), and so on. Whenever a noun or pronoun's semantic function is unclear in this way, the term Entity is used, and 2-element combinations classified accordingly:

Ent + Ent *that a ball, he doctor* (a major construction for indicating identification or classification), *mummy daddy*
Ent + Attr *that nice, the man happy*
Ent + Temp *man now, ice-cream in minute*
Ent + Loc *man there, chair on floor*
Ent + Other *man no, car to*

Again, element order is not significant: *man now* and *now man* are both Ent + Temp. (But it should be noted that many examples of Attr + Ent will be indistinguishable from the Stage I construction Entity (with Attribute specification), e.g. *happy man, nice car*. Unless there is clear evidence of a 2-element clause, these should be classified at Stage I.)

Lastly, a section is included to handle other combinations which do not fall into the main types named above: Other + Other, e.g. *there in garden* (Loc + Loc), *quickly now* (Manner + Temp).

Any cooccurring specifications of these elements are classified using the same general procedure as at Stage I. For example, *man go* is Act + Dyn, and here there are no specifications; *the man is going* is also Act + Dyn, but in this case a mark would be placed opposite Definiteness in the Actor column, and opposite Other in the Dynamic column. Other examples of this kind are:

Sentence	Elements	Specification
two people came	Act Dyn	Quantity (in Act column)
gone in garden	Dyn Loc	Scope (in Loc column)
that man a doctor	Ent Ent	Definiteness (in Ent column) twice
my cow has jumped	Act Dyn	Possessive (in Act column) Other (in Dyn column)

Two other points are routinely noted at Stage II. First, the occurrence of interrogative words as elements of clause structure is noted, *in addition* to their function as Actor, Goal, Locative, or whatever. For example, in the clause *where going,* we have Loc + Dyn, and this would be noted in the appropriate box. But in addition, a mark would be placed under +*Interr,* enabling us to see developments in this specific semantic area. Secondly, the use of deictic forms as elements of clause structure continues to be monitored: any occurrence of a deictic is noted in the relevant box, *in addition* to being analysed for its clausal function above. For example, *man there* is Ent + Loc, and this would be noted in the appropriate box. A mark would also be placed in the Deictic box in the Loc column, representing the item *there.*

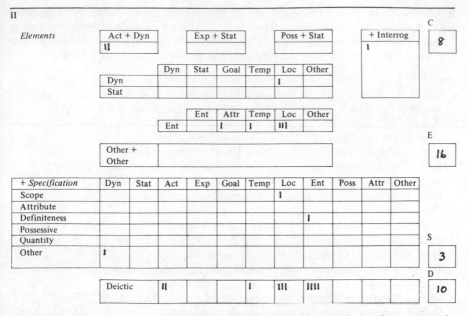

Lastly, it should be noted that the copula, having no independent semantic function, is not included as a semantic clause element. Thus, *the man is in the garden* is analysed as a 2-element clause (Ent + Loc), and likewise *where is the car* (Loc + Ent), *that is a cat* (Ent + Ent), and so on. Similarly, 'empty' *it* and *there* are ignored, e.g. *it's a man running* is analysed as Act + Dyn (the same as *a man is running*), *there's a cow in the garden* is Ent + Loc, and so on. The same procedure is followed in later Stages.

The totalling procedure is the same as for Stage 1, except for the distinction which must now be made between *number of clauses* (C) and *number of clause elements* (E); the significance of this distinction is indicated in 5.9.7. Total specifications and total deictic forms are provided.

The following set of Stage II sentences was taken from a language-delayed child of 4, and analysed as shown to produce the profile below. The reliance on a few clausal combinations—especially involving Locative—the absence of specifications, and a marked deictic bias should be noted.

Sentence	Element	Specification	
man in there	Ent Loc	Scope (Loc)	Deic
him fallen	Act Dyn	—	Deic
that one there	Ent Loc	Definite (Ent)	Deic (× 2)
put – in	Dyn Loc	—	Deic
that nice	Ent Attr	—	Deic
where that	Loc Ent	—	Deic
			Interr
me now	Ent Temp	—	Deic (× 2)
he isn't			
(i.e. jumping)	Act Dyn	Other (Dyn)	Deic

5.9.5 Stage II clauses consist of 3 major semantic elements, classified according to the functions listed in 5.9.2. At this point in development, a wide range of semantic combinations is possible. Five important combinations are specified on the chart, but a large space is available for Other types.

Act + Dyn + Goal	*the man is kicking the ball*
Act + Dyn + Temp	*the man is running already*
Act + Dyn + Loc	*the man is running into the street*
Act + Dyn + Other	*the man is running quickly* (Manner)
Exp + Stat + Goal	*the man sees a ball*
Exp + Stat + Temp	*the man is trying now*
Exp + Stat + Loc	*the man can see around the corner*
Exp + Stat + Other	*the man seems nice* (Attribute)
Poss + Stat + Goal	*the man has got a car*
Poss + Stat + Temp	*you have now*
Poss + Stat + Loc	*you have there*
Poss + Stat + Other	*you have big* (Attribute)
Dyn + Goal + Goal	*give me a letter*
Dyn + Goal + Temp	*kicked the ball then*
Dyn + Goal + Loc	*put the ball there*
Dyn + Goal + Other	*put the ball carefully*
Stat + Goal + Goal	*wish you luck*
Stat + Goal + Temp	*saw him the next day*
Stat + Goal + Loc	*saw him there*
Stat + Goal + Other	*thought him nice* (Attribute)

Other combinations include: Ent + Ent + Temp *the man a ball now*
Dyn + Loc + Temp *go there now*
Ent + Loc + Loc *a man there in the garden*
etc.

As with the previous Stage, the order of elements is not significant, specifications are noted in the appropriate columns as they occur, deictics and interrogatives are given additional marks, and totals are indicated in the right-hand margin. The following examples are illustrative:

Sentence	Elements	Specification
the man kicked my car	Act Dyn Goal	Definiteness (Act) Possessive (Goal)
he has three eggs	Poss Stat Goal	Quantity (Goal) Deictic (Poss)
he is happy there	Ent Attr Loc	Deictic (Other) Deictic (Loc)
	(copula not being included as a semantic element)	
who saw the box	Exp Stat Goal	Definiteness (Goal) + Interr

These 4 sentences would transfer onto the Stage III section of the chart in the following way.

III

Elements	+ Goal	+ Temp	+ Loc	+ Other
Act + Dyn	I			
Exp + Stat	I			
Poss + Stat	I			
Dyn + Goal				
Stat + Goal				
Other	Ent + Attr + Loc I			

+ Interrog	C
I	4

E 12

+ Specification	Dyn	Stat	Act	Exp	Poss	Goal	Temp	Loc	Other
Scope									
Attribute									
Definiteness			I		I				
Possessive					I				
Quantity					I				
Other									
Deictic				I				I	I

S 4

D 3

5.9.6 Stage IV clauses consist of four or more semantic elements, classified according to the functions listed in 5.9.2. Once again, in view of the wide range of possible combinations, only the most central types can be individually named, as follows:

Act+Dyn+Goal+Temp   *the man is kicking the ball now*
Act+Dyn+Goal+Loc   *the man is kicking the ball into the goal*
Act+Dyn+Goal+Other   *the man is kicking the ball hard* (Manner)
Exp+Stat+Goal+Temp   *the man saw me yesterday*
Exp+Stat+Goal +Loc   *the man saw me in the garden*
Exp+Stat+Goal+Other   *the man wanted me ready* (Attribute)
Poss+Stat+Goal+Temp   *he has a car now*
Poss+Stat+Goal+Loc   *he has a car in the garage*
Poss+Stat+Goal+Other   *he has a car for me* (Benefactive)
Other combinations include   Act+Dyn+Loc+Temp   *he went home yesterday*

Dyn+Goal+Loc+Loc   *kicked the ball over the wall and into the field*

etc.

As with the previous Stage, the order of elements is not significant, specifications are noted in the appropriate columns as they occur, deictics and interrogatives are given additional marks, and totals are indicated in the right-hand margin. The following examples are illustrative:

Sentence	Elements	Specification	
the man saw me there	Exp Stat Goal Loc	Definiteness (Exp)	Deictic (Goal)
			Deictic (Loc)
I like eating eggs	Exp Stat Dyn Goal	—	Deictic (Exp)
two men turned the	Act Dyn Goal Other	Quantity (Act)	
* wheel slowly*		Definiteness (Goal)	

These three sentences would transfer onto the Stage IV section of the chart in the following way:

IV

Elements	+ Temp	+ Loc	+ Other		+ Interrog	C
Act + Dyn + Goal						**3**
Exp + Stat + Goal		I				
Poss + Stat + Goal						E
Other	Exp + Stat + Dyn + Goal I					**12**
	Act + Dyn + Goal + Other I					

+ Specification	Dyn	Stat	Act	Exp	Poss	Goal	Temp	Loc	Other	
Scope										
Attribute										
Definiteness			I			I				
Possessive										
Quantity			I							S
Other										**3**
										D
Deictic				I		I		I		**3**

It is impracticable to specify the wide range of clauses containing 5 or more semantic elements. The section is thus left blank, to be filled in as need arises. Nor is it possible to specify deictics and specifications in detail. Thus, for example, the clause *John saw me in town yesterday* (Exp + Stat + Goal + Loc + Temp) would be listed in the 5+ section, along with a mark under deictic (for *me*) and one under specification (for *in*), as follows:

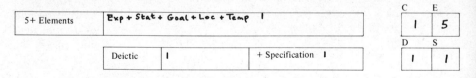

5+ Elements	Exp + Stat + Goal + Loc + Temp I	C	E
		I	**5**
		D	S
Deictic I	+ Specification I	**I**	**I**

5.9.7 A selection of useful quantitative measures is given at the foot of page 2 of the PRISM-G chart:

the total number of major clauses is obtained by adding the totals in the boxes marked C in the right-hand columns of pages 1 and 2;
the total number of clause elements is obtained by adding the totals in the boxes marked E in these margins;

the total number of specifications is obtained by adding the totals in the boxes marked S in these columns;
the total number of deictics is obtained by adding the totals in the boxes marked D in these columns.

Various ratios can now be obtained, of which the most important seem to be:

mean number of elements per clause (Total E divided by Total C);
mean number of specifications per element (Total S divided by Total E);
mean number of deictics per clause element (Total D divided by Total E).

An example of this procedure is given in 5.10.

5.9.8 Stage V deals with the semantic relationships between clauses occurring within the same sentence.

The clearest cases are coordination sequences. Here the first clause is taken as a given, the second clause related to the first, the third (if there is one) to the second, and so on, as follows:

Clause 1 +Clause 2
        Clause 2 + Clause 3
                Clause 3 + Clause 4
                        etc.

For example, in the sentence *John kicked the ball and Mary caught it and Mike laughed,* the relationship between the first two clauses would be noted (using the Connective *and,* in its function of Addition), and then the relationship between the second and third (Addition again).

For sentences involving grammatical subordination, the procedure is slightly more complex, as two levels of analysis are involved. It is no longer a simple matter of sequence, but of the simultaneous processing of clauses. When the subordinate clause expresses the *whole* of a clause element, the semantic role of the whole clause is first noted, in relation to the main clause, in the manner already described for Stages I to IV; then the internal semantic structure of the subordinate clause is analysed—also in terms of Stages I to IV. For example, in the sentence *he came when John waved,* we have an adverbial clause of time. The first level of analysis is therefore Act + Dyn + Temp. The Temp element is then analysed in terms of its own clause structure, as Connective + Act + Dyn. The two stages can be summarized most clearly in the following way:

he came when John waved
Act Dyn   Temp   (Stage III)
        ┌────────┴────────┐
        Conn Act   Dyn   (Stage II)

Each of these structures would be noted at the appropriate Stage (along with any deictics/specifications). At Stage V, then, it remains only to note that a sequence has occurred, and what kind of sequence it is (see further below).

A similar procedure is used for cases where the subordinate clause expresses only a *part* of a clause element—as when nouns are postmodified.

Here, the superordinate clause is analysed in the usual way, and the subordinate clause then analysed in its own terms, as follows:

the man I saw kicked the ball

Superordinate clause	Act	Dyn	Goal	(Stage III)
Subordinate clause	Exp Stat			(Stage II)

Each of these structures would be noted at the appropriate Stage (along with any deictics/specifications). The fact of the sequence would then be noted at Stage V (see further below).

It should be noted that the use of relative pronouns poses an analysis problem—whether to take the relative pronoun as Connective or as a clause element in its own right (Act, Goal etc.). For example, in the sentence *the man whom I saw . . . ,* it would be possible to see *whom* as Connective, or to analyse it as Goal to the verb *saw;* similarly with *the place where I went* (with *where* being Loc to the verb *went*), and so on. The present procedure adopts the former alternative (as does the LARSP chart: see 2.13.3).

One further analytic problem should be mentioned: the case of sentences such as *he wanted the man to go.* Again, to be consistent with LARSP, these sentences are analysed as single clauses. Because *the man* is both part of the Goal of *wanted* and at the same time the Actor for *go,* an analysis of Entity is made. The structure of this sentence is therefore: Exp + Stat + Ent + Dyn— that is, a Stage IV structure.

5.9.9 The matrix at Stage V provides an initial classification of the type of semantic relationship which links successive clauses, and an indication of the relative complexity (measured in terms of number of semantic elements) of the clauses in the sequence.

Eight types of semantic relationship are recognized, as follows:

Addition   typically, the use of *and,* e.g. *John came and I did too;*
Reformulation   typically, the use of *or,* e.g. *we sang or they danced;*
Contrast   typically, the use of *but,* e.g. *he called but I was out;*
Temporal   typically, the use of *when, after, before, while,* e.g. *he came after I left;*
Cause   typically, the use of *because, since, as,* e.g. *he cried 'cos he fell;*
Location   typically *where, wherever,* e.g. *he asked where I was;*
Condition   typically *if, (al)though, unless, whether,* e.g. *if it falls, it will break;*
Purpose   typically, *(in order) to, (so as) to, so (that),* e.g. *he came so I left;*
Other   including *as* (= 'how'), *rather, than, seeing that, as if, as though,* and the relative pronouns. Tag questions, tag statements, comment clauses, etc. (no connectives involved) are also logged under Other, e.g. *that's John; isn't it; that's John, that is; that's John, you know.*

It should be noted that some items have variable function, depending on context: this is especially the case with *and,* which is sometimes used in temporal or purposive function (e.g. *he came and (so) I left, we went to the shops and (then) bought a coat*).

Under these headings, each subordinate or coordinated clause is identified in terms of whether a connective is present or absent. In most sequences in normal adult English, connectives are obligatory; but in clinical settings, omitted connectives are common. For example, P might say *he asked I was,* meaning 'he asked where I was': this would be logged under the heading Location (which is the intended function of the subordinate clause), and under $\emptyset$ (i.e. 'zero connective'). The same principle applies to all the other categories.

The vertical dimension of the Stage V matrix enables us to indicate the relative complexity of any pair of clauses, using the (admittedly crude) index of the number of semantic elements the clauses contain. For example, 2 + 2 would mean that P had used a combination of 2 clauses, each containing 2 elements (e.g. *John ran and I walked*), 3 + 1 would refer to a sequence in which the first clause had three elements and the second had only one (e.g. *John kicked the ball and goal*). In subordinate clause relationships, one counts the main clause elements first, and then the subordinate clause (e.g. *he came when I left* . . . is analysed as 3 + 2); a subsequent coordinate clause would be related to the previous main clause (e.g. . . . *and saw the dog* would be 3 + 2). The set of possibilities recognized in the left-hand column are:

1 + 1, 1 + 2, 1 + 3$^+$ (i.e. the second clause contains 3 or more elements)
2 + 1, 2 + 2, 2 + 3$^+$
3 + 1, 3 + 2, 3 + 3$^+$
4$^+$ + 1, 4$^+$ + 2, 4$^+$ + 3$^+$ (i.e. the first clause contains 4 or more elements and the second clause contains 3 or more elements)

The clinical expectation, of course, is that P's ability to develop his use of clause sequences will be partly dependent on the amount of semantic information each clause (especially the first in a sequence) contains. Problems of memory and attention, in particular, will affect his ability to produce balanced sequences of multi-element clauses.

As errors in developing good clause sequences are a particular problem area in assessment and remediation, one further factor is introduced into the matrix—namely, whether P's sequence is acceptable or unacceptable (indicated by $\sqrt{}$ and X respectively). The final layout of the matrix is thus as follows:

Clause (A–B) Sequence

		Addition		Reform.		Contrast		Temporal		Cause		Location		Condition		Purpose		Other	
		Conn	φ	Conn	φ	Conn	φ	Conn	φ	Conn	φ	Conn	φ	Conn	φ	Conn	φ	Conn	φ
$1 + 1$	√																		
	×																		
$1 + 2$	√																		
	×																		
$1 + 3^+$	√																		
	×																		
$2 + 1$	√																		
	×																		
$2 + 2$	√																		
	×																		
$2 + 3^+$	√																		
	×																		
$3 + 1$	√																		
	×																		
$3 + 2$	√																		
	×																		
$3 + 3^+$	√																		
	×																		
$4^+ + 1$	√																		
	×																		
$4^+ + 2$	√																		
	×																		
$4^+ + 3^+$	√																		
	×																		

We can see the way in which these various factors intersect by applying the procedure to the following examples:

Sentence	Semantic Relationships	Connective Present	No. of Elements	√ or X	Matrix Location
he laughed and I laughed	Addition	Conn.	$2 + 2$	√	see below

Matrix Location detail:

	Addition	
	Conn	φ
$2 + 2$ √	I	
×		

Sentence	Semantic Relationships	Connective Present	No. of Elements	√ or X	Matrix Location
I saw the man when he arrived	Temporal	Conn.	4 + 2	√	Temporal: Conn / φ ... 4 + 2 √ 1 / X
me want that cos it big	Cause	Conn.	4 + 2	√	Cause: Conn / φ ... 4 + 2 √ 1 / X
the ladder slip cos my arm broke	Cause	Conn.	3 + 2	X	Cause: Conn / φ ... 3 + 2 √ / X 1

Sentence	Semantic Relationships	Connective Present	No. of Elements	√ or X	Matrix Location
he know what him write	Other	Conn.	3 + 2	√	Other

					Conn	φ
				3 + 2	√	I	
					X		

| *he hurt his arm while he fell* | Temporal | Conn. | 4 + 2 | X | Temporal |

					Conn	φ
				4 + 2	√		
					X	I	

| *that's the place I like* | Other | Ø | 2 + 2 | √ | Other |

					Conn	φ
				2 + 2	√		I
					X		

Sentence	Semantic Relationships	Connective Present	No. of Elements	√ or X	Matrix Location
he falls he'll be hurt	Condition	Ø	2 + 2	X	Condition / Conn φ
			2 + 2	√	
				X	I

It is often the case that, as P attempts to sequence clauses, he produces many sequences which are ambiguous, incoherent, incomplete, etc. Clause pairs which are not analysed, for whatever reason, are marked under the heading Unanalysed at the top of the Stage V section. For example, *the man has – er – has – and got a man lots* looks as if it might be a 2-clause sequence, but the incompleteness of the first clause, and the uncertain word order of the second would make this a candidate for Unanalysed. Similarly, *he kick the ball got ball* (said within a single intonation contour) seems to be an attempt at a 2-clause sentence (as opposed to two separate sentences), but it is unclear which semantic relation is being expressed (= 'he kicked the ball when he received the ball'? 'he kicked the ball and so someone else received the ball'? etc.). The total under Unanalysed will often be an important indication of P's progress in handling clause sequencing.

5.9.10 Two other kinds of sequencing information are routinely recorded in Stage V. (This by no means exhausts the range of semantic factors which might be taken into account in an analysis of discourse; they are simply two factors whose clinical usefulness has often been noted.)

(a) The *order-of-mention* of clauses in a sentence is noted, i.e. whether the order in which the clauses appear corresponds to the order of events in the world. The simplest state of affairs is for the linguistic 'events' and the real world events to be in parallel, e.g. in the sentence *I got up and went to the window,* the first event which took place was the getting up, and this was the subject-matter of the first clause; the second event which took place was the subject-matter of the second clause. Language permits various departures from this norm, however, and these may pose problems for P, both in comprehension and production. For example, *I got up after I went to the window* reverses the order-of-mention, as the first clause expresses the event which took place second. Ps have particular difficulty understanding such reversals (e.g. in instruction tasks of the kind 'Do X after you do Y' or 'Before you do X, do Y'), and the stage at which they introduce such reversals accurately into their own speech indicates an important piece of semantic learning.

Five order-of-mention possibilities are recognized on the PRISM-G chart at Stage V:

$C_1 \rightarrow C_2$ i.e. the order of the 2 clauses in a sentence preserves order-of-mention, as in *I got up and went to the window;*

$C_1 \rightarrow C_2 \rightarrow C_3$ i.e. the order of 3 clauses in a sentence preserves order-of-mention, e.g. *I got up, went to the window, and looked out;*

Other → i.e. any longer sequence which preserves order-of-mention;

$C_2 \leftarrow C_1$ i.e. the order of the 2 clauses reverses order-of-mention, as in *I got up after I went to the window;*

Other ← i.e. any longer sequence in which order-of-mention is not preserved, e.g. *before you go outside to play, I want you to be quiet and first put your books away* (a genuine classroom example!).

In each case, the possibility has to be anticipated that the clause sequence, in whichever order, is correct or incorrect. For example, one P said *he went fishing and saw a bus* (referring to a picture sequence). If he was describing a picture sequence where Picture 1 showed a man going fishing, and Picture 2 showed a bus, then the use of this connective would correctly relate the 2 clauses to the 2 events. But if the pictures had been the other way round, P's version would (in the context of the task) be incorrect. The chart thus has to allow for the correct use of a $C_1 \rightarrow C_2$ sequence, and its incorrect use, and this is done by using $\sqrt{}$ and X. Similarly, if P said *before he went fishing he saw a bus,* this could be a correct use of a connective marking reversed order-of-mention sentence, or an incorrect one, depending on the way in which the pictures were actually presented. Once again, therefore, the $\sqrt{}$/X distinction is needed—and it is in fact used for all the categories in this section of the chart.

(b) The study of the semantics of discourse interaction is in its infancy, hence only a token statement can be made about this area on a chart of this kind. The central issue is the extent to which we can capture P's ability to produce semantically self-contained clauses, as opposed to his being dependent on T's stimuli. Both the following single-element clauses would be labelled Loc in the above approach, for example:

P (*picking up a toy*) hère/   T 'where are you góing/
                                  P 'over thère/

They would both be classified in the appropriate boxes in Stage I. But this would be to miss the point that *over there* has a specific semantic relation to the semantic structure of T's stimulus—and might perhaps have been expanded into *you're going over there* by T subsequently. A section has therefore been added to Stage V (though it is by no means clear that this is the best place to put it) in which the analyst can indicate how many and which kind of semantic elements in T's stimulus P is taking for granted in this way. P might take just a single element for granted, or 2 or more elements from a clause—or even a whole clause. The main possibilities are given at the foot of page 3, under the heading *Presupposed T elements*, as follows:

Act/Exp presupposed, e.g.
    T 'where's the màn/
    P 'walking in the gàrden/ (*the man/he* presupposed)

Dyn/Stat presupposed, e.g.

T   'what's the 'man kìcking/
P   'man a bàll/ (*kicking* presupposed)

Goal presupposed, e.g.

T   did he 'kick the báll/
P   he dìd 'kick/ (*the ball* presupposed)

Scope presupposed, e.g.

T   the 'man's in the gàrden/ ìsn't he/
P   yès/ he ìs/ (*in the garden* presupposed)

Other element (e.g. Entity) or part of element presupposed, e.g.

T   'how many rùns did you 'get/
P   I 'got tèn/ (*runs* presupposed, but this is only part of the element Goal)

2 elements presupposed, e.g.

T   'where's the càr 'gone/
P   'into the gàrage/ (*the car* and *gone* presupposed)

3 or more elements presupposed, within a single clause, e.g.

T   'where has 'John 'put the létter/
P   in his pòcket/ (*John*, *put* and *letter* presupposed)

Whole clause presupposed, e.g.

T   'why did you 'do thàt/
P   'cos I wànted to/ (*I did that* presupposed)

The √/X distinction once again needs to be invoked. It is possible for P to presuppose one or more elements correctly or incorrectly. In all the examples above, P has made intelligible assumptions in what he has said: in each case, T's sentence fills the gaps in P's utterance. But in the following cases, this does not happen:

T   'what can you 'see in the pìcture/
P   wàlking/ (i.e. Act presupposed, but incorrectly, which leads T to say)
T   whò is/

. . .

T   'what's the 'man dóing/
P   'man – in a trèe/ (i.e. probably Dyn presupposed, e.g. *climbing*, but this is semantically unacceptable, given the open question stimulus)

When it is plain that P is presupposing an element (or elements) in T's stimulus for which there is no justification, the point is noted along the X line of this section.

These remaining sections of Stage V are laid out on the chart as follows:

Order-of-mention

	$C_1 \rightarrow C_2$	$C_1 \rightarrow C_2 \rightarrow C_3$	Other $\rightarrow$	$C_2 \leftarrow C_1$	Other $\leftarrow$
√					
×					

Presupposed T elements

	1					2	3+	Clause
	Act/Exp	Dyn/Stat	Goal	Scope	Other			
√								
×								

Idiomatic

Error

5.9.11 There are two remaining observations to make about the application of the PRISM-G procedure. Firstly, in the course of analysis, one will encounter sentences which defy semantic analysis in conventional terms, because of their idiomatic (or partly idiomatic) character. For example, a sentence such as *I take pleasure in reading* begins plainly enough, with Exp— but how to analyse *take pleasure?* It is hardly *take + pleasure*. Until such time as adequate typologies of idiomatic structures become available, all one can do is list such examples as they occur, and a section of the chart (at the foot of page 3) has been left for the purpose (headed *Idiomatic*). It is important to note that the *whole* of any sentence placed into this section is left unanalysed.

Secondly, in the course of analysis, one will encounter sentences which seem to be semantic errors, in the sense that it proves impossible to assign a coherent interpretation to the sentence, using the language provided. For example, one P said *see a man and a garage go*. This is 'plainly' Stat + Ent + Ent + Dyn. It is not clear whether the Entities are Act, Exp, Loc, Other, or whatever. Perhaps one day we may dare to call such sequences deviant. For the moment, they are simply listed in full, under the heading of Error at the foot of page 3 of the chart.

5.10 It will be evident from the above that the two subprocedures, PRISM-L and PRISM-G, are independently constructed, and it is perfectly in order to use one of the procedures without the other. On the other hand, as already pointed out (5.2), the information each provides needs to be placed in the context of the other, before a full semantic interpretation can be arrived at. To know that P uses an item such as *horse* is only half the story; it is also important to know whether he can use it as Actor, Goal, Locative, and so on. One frequently encounters Ps who can use an item in one semantic role but not in another. Conversely, to note the occurrence of a particular semantic construction (say, Act + Dyn + Goal) is one thing; it is also important to know whether each of these elements can be used with a good lexical range. One frequently encounters Ps for whom a semantic role is expressed only by one or two lexemes (e.g. Dyn can only be *go* or *do*). Wherever possible, therefore, we use both procedures on samples.

The above account, it is hoped, will anticipate the majority of the semantic features encountered in clinical samples. Problematic items and patterns are only to be expected, though, given the lack of research into semantic typology, and the well-known difficulties of arriving at satisfactory contextual interpretations. Often one feels reasonably confident about an analytic decision, but lacks total certainty; we indicate such problem items/sentences with question-marks (as will be illustrated below), and they deserve separate study. Often the analyst's uncertainty reflects a difficulty on the part of the patient.

The following short extract illustrates the two PRISM procedures in use with a 55-year-old dysphasic man. The sample is taken from the beginning of a session, but is not thereby atypical: the strategies P uses here are found throughout the session, regardless of topic or task. The account is given in three stages. For each sentence in the sample, a corresponding analysis is made in terms of PRISM-L (first column) and PRISM-G (second column): for the PRISM-L analysis, each item in the sentence is taken in order, and its place identified on the chart; for the PRISM-G analysis, the relevant Stage is first identified, along with details of the semantic elements involved, and this is followed by details of Specifications (if any), Deictics (if any), and information about Stage V (if any). Following the analysis, the relevant sections of the PRISM-L chart, and the whole of the PRISM-G chart, are printed, with the items and patterns filled in. Finally, a brief discussion of the main patterns follows.

		PRISM-L	*PRISM-G*
T	'like to sit thére/		
P	àh/	Minor: Social Response	I Social Minor
	thànk you/ --	Minor: Social Response	I Social Minor
T	'how did you gèt here to'day/		
P	òh/	Minor: Social Response	I Social Minor
	'just wàlked/ .	State (Intensity)	II Dyn + Other
		Moving (Animate)	V Act presupposed √
	I 'only gò 'round the córner/	Minor: Pronominal 1	III Act + Dyn + Loc
		State (Intensity)	Specifications:
		Moving (Come/Go)	Sco (Loc)
		Minor: Prepositional (Loc)	Def (Loc)
			Oth (Loc)
		Minor: Pronominal (Art)	Deic (Act)
		Location (General)	
T	'oh I sèe/		
P	'only 'just r. 'round hère/	State (Intensity)	I Deic (Sco)
		State (Intensity)	Specifications:
		Minor: Prepositional (Loc)	Oth (Sco)
			Oth (Sco)
		Location (General)	Sco (Sco)

		PRISM-L	*PRISM-G*
T	òh/		V Act + Dyn presupposed √
	so *it's 'very hăndy/		
P	*so	Minor: Connective	Incomplete
	yès/	Minor: Social	I Social Minor
		Response	
	'very . 'very gòod/ –	State (Intensity)	I Attr
		State (Quality)	Specifications:
		(the first use of *very*	Oth (Attr)
		is discounted, as	
		nonfluency)	V ?Ent presupposed √
T	'so you could wălk/		
P	wèll/	Minor: Social	I Social Minor
		Response	
	yès/	Minor: Social	I Social Minor
		Response	
	I 'only wàlked a'bout 'two .	Minor: Pronominal 1	III Act + Dyn + Temp
	'three mínutes *and	State (Intensity)	Specifications:
	I'm bàck/	Moving (Animate)	Qua (Temp)
		(repeat)	Qua (Temp)
		Minor: Prepositional	Sco (Temp)
		(Temp)	Oth (Temp)
		Quantity (Specific)	Deic (Act)
		Quantity (Specific)	II Exp + Loc
		Measurement (Time)	Deic (Exp)
		Minor: Connective	Deic (Loc)
		Minor: Pronominal 1	V Temp
		Minor: Verbal (be)	3 + 2
		Location (General)	Conn √
T	*oh I sèe/		Order-of-mention
	oh 'that's vêry 'good/		C1 → C2 √
P	yès/ yès/ yès/ yès/ . yès/	Minor: Social	I Social Minor (×5)
		Response (×5)	
T	so . 'did you 'get wèt/		
P	nò/ .	Minor: Social	I Social Minor
		Response	
	nò/ .	Minor: Social	I Social Minor
		Response	
	it [s] it sèemed/ . 'just	Minor: Empty	Ambiguous
	a'bout a 'whole 'lot of [l]	(first *it* nonfluent)	
	a 'bit lŏnger/ but it 'looks	Thinking (Process)	(a) relation of *a*
	as 'though it mìght 'be	State (Intensity)	*whole lot of* to the
	agáin/ *and 'I shan't	Minor: Prepositional	rest of the first
		(Temp)	clause unclear;
		Minor: Pronominal (Art)	(b) unclear what kind
		State (Intensity)	of verb omitted in
		Quantity (General)	second clause;
		Minor: Prepositional	(c) third clause
		(Other)	incomplete
		Minor: Pronominal (Art)	(d) *longer, be*—unclear
		Quantity (General)	presuppositions
		Time (Period)	
		Minor: Connective	
		Minor: Empty	
		Sight (Act) +	
		[Thinking(Process)]	
		Minor: Connective	

		PRISM-L	PRISM-G
		Minor: Empty	
		Minor: Verbal (Other)	
		Minor: Verbal (be)	
		Time (Frequency)	
		Minor: Connective	
		Minor: Pronominal 1	
		Minor: Verbal (Neg)	
T	*it dòes/ dòesn't it/ m̀/		
P	yèah/ . yèah/ . yèah/ . yèah/	Minor: Social Response (×4)	I Social Minor (×4)
T	you 'might 'catch it 'going hŏme/		
P	wèll/	Minor: Social Response	I Social Minor
	I mìght 'do/	Minor: Pronominal 1	II Exp + Stat (?)
		Minor: Verbal (Other)	Specifications:
		Minor: Verbal (Other)	Oth (Stat)
			Deic (Exp)
			V Goal + Loc presupposed √
	I'll 'have to sèe/ (*laughs*)	Minor: Pronominal 1	II Exp + Stat
		Minor: Verbal (Other)	Specifications:
		Minor: Verbal (Other)	Oth (Stat)
		Sight (Act)	Oth (Stat)
			Deic (Exp)
T	'what do you thìnk of the 'weather/ – *we've been hàving/		
P	*wèll/	Minor: Social Reponse	I Social Minor
	it's 'been 'very bàd/ up to nǒw/	Minor: Pronominal 3	III Ent + Attr + Temp
		Minor: Verbal (Other)	Specifications:
		Minor: Verbal (be)	Oth (Other)
		State (Intensity)	Sco (Temp)
		State (Quality)	Deic (Other)
		Minor: Prepositional (Temp)	Deic (Temp)
		Time (Present)	
T	*m̀/		
P	*there 'was a'bout 'three ooh a 'bit lònger than thát/	Minor: Empty	Ambiguous
		Minor: Verbal (be)	
		Minor: Prepositional (Temp)	(a) The clause changes direction mid-way
		Quantity (Specific)	(b) Unclear presuppositions
		Minor: Social Spontaneous	(*longer, that*)
		Minor: Pronominal (Art)	
		Quantity (General)	
		Measurement (Time)	
		Minor: Connective	
		Minor: Pronominal (Dem)	
	it was 'very gǒod/	Minor: Pronominal 3	II Ent + Attr
		Minor: Verbal (be)	Specifications:
		State (Intensity)	Oth (Attr)
		State (Quality)	Deic (Ent)
T	yèah/ . *'that's rìght/		

		PRISM-L	PRISM-G
P	*but . but ŏtherwise/ nò/	Minor: Connective (first *but* nonfluent) State (Like −) Minor: Social Spon- taneous	I Social Minor Specifications (×2) V presupposed clause X
T	been àwful/ hàsn't it/		
P	yèah/	Minor: Social Response	I Social Minor
	wèll/ .	Minor: Social Response	I Social Minor
	'there you àre/	Minor: Stereotype	I Other Minor
	it's the 'sort of 'thing	Minor: Empty	III Act + Dyn + Goal
	you 'have to lèave .	Minor: Verbal (be)	(i.e. *you + have to*
	you sée/	Minor: Pronominal (Art) State (Like +) Other Minor: Pronominal 3 (= 'one') Minor: Verbal (Other) Moving (Come/Go) Minor: Comment	*leave + the sort of* *thing*) Specifications: Oth (Dyn) Def (Goal) ?Oth (Goal) (*sort of*) I Other Minor V Other 3 + 1 ∅ √
T	yès/ in 'this cóuntry/		
P	er . I I've . 'been lătely/ . 'doing 'things mysèlf/ . er with	(first *I* nonfluent) Minor: Pronominal 1 Minor: Verbal (Other) Minor: Verbal (be) Time (Past) Making/Doing (General) Other Minor: Pronominal 1 Minor: Prepositional (Prob)	IV Act + Dyn + Goal + Temp Specifications: Oth (Dyn) Oth (Dyn) Oth (Act) (*myself*) Deic (Act) (×2) (the *with* construction is left incomplete, but the final intonation of the first clause, and the
T	păinting/		intervening pause, gives it the appearance of an afterthought)
P	yès/ .	Minor: Social Response	I Social Minor
	'and (4 sylls)	Minor: Connective Unintelligible	Unintelligible
	it will be 'three wèeks it will 'be álmost/	Minor: Empty Minor: Verbal (Other) Minor: Verbal (be) Quantity (Specific) Measurement (Time) Minor: Empty Minor: Verbal (Other) Minor: Verbal (*be*) State (Like +)	II Temp + Temp Specifications: Qua (Temp) V Presupposed clause X
T	(my) gòodness/ is 'that 'outsĭde/		

		PRISM-L	PRISM-G
P	nò/	Minor: Social Response	I Social Minor
	*ìnside/	Location (Specific)	I Deic (Sco)
T	*ìnside/		
P	nò/	Minor: Social Response	I Social Minor
	it's 'too ['bɑ] bàd to 'do 'anything élse/ .	Minor: Pronominal 3 (i.e. the weather)	II Ent + Attr Specifications:
		Minor: Verbal (be)	Oth (Attr)
		State (Intensity)	Deic (Ent)
		State (Quality)	II Dyn + Goal
		Minor: Empty	Specifications:
		Making/Doing (General)	Oth (Goal) (*else*)
		Other	Deic (Goal)
		Quantity (General)	V Other
			2 + 2
			Ø √
	'all the 'other 'things 'seem to fínish/ . so I 'thought well I'll 'go and dò it/ – and it's 'not 'too bád/ réally/	Quantity (General)	III Goal + Stat + Dyn
		Minor: Pronominal (Art)	(i.e. 'seem to be
		Quantity (General)	finished')
		Other	Specifications:
		Thinking (Process)	Qua (Goal)
		Minor: Empty	Def (Goal)
		Happening	Attr (Goal)
		Minor: Connective	Deic (Goal)
		Minor: Pronominal 1	III Exp + Stat + Goal
		Thinking (Process)	
		Minor: Social Spon- tancous	IV Act + Dyn + Dyn + Goal
		Minor: Pronominal 1	(I Social minor) (*well*)
		Minor: Verbal (Other)	Specifications:
		Moving (Come/Go)	Oth (Dyn) ('*ll*)
		Minor: Connective	Oth (Dyn) (*and*)
		Making/Doing (General)	Deic (Exp) (at III)
		Minor: Pronominal 3	Deic (Act) (at IV)
		Minor: Connective	Deic (Goal) (at IV)
		Minor: Pronominal 3	II Ent + Attr
		Minor: Verbal (*be*)	Specifications:
		Minor: Verbal (Neg)	Oth (Attr)
		State (Intensity)	Oth (Attr)
		State (Quality)	Deic (Ent)
		Minor: Comment	I Other Minor (*really*)
			V Purpose
			3 + 3
			Conn √
			V Other
			3 + 3+
			Ø √
			V Addition
			3 + 2
			Conn √
			V other
			2 + 1
			Ø √

		PRISM-L	PRISM-G
T	yès/ . gòod/		Order-of-mention C1 → C2 → C3 √
P	I . I 'haven't . dòne it/ for . 'three yĕars/	(first *I* nonfluent) Minor: Pronominal 1 Minor: Verbal (Neg) Making/Doing (General) Minor: Pronominal 3 Minor: Prepositional (Temp) Quantity (Specific) Measurement (Time)	IV Act + Dyn + Goal + Temp Specifications: Oth (Dyn) (*have*) Oth (Dyn) (*n't*) Sco (Temp) Qua (Temp) Deic (Act) Deic (Goal)
T	*nò/		
P	*sò/ I thòught/ I'll 'go and 'see how it ìs/	Minor: Connective Minor: Pronominal 1 Thinking (Process) Minor: Pronominal 1 Minor: Verbal (Other) Moving (Come/Go) Minor: Connective Sight (Act) Minor: Connective Minor: Pronominal 3 Happening (?)	III Exp + Stat + Goal IV Act + Dyn + Stat + Goal II Exp + Stat(?) Specifications: Oth (Dyn) (at III) Oth (Stat) (at III) Deic (Exp) (at III) Deic (Act) (at IV) Deic (Exp) (at II)
T	*m̀/		
P	*and I 'think it is 'better than it wàs/	Minor: Connective Minor: Pronominal 1 Thinking (Process) Minor: Pronominal 3 Minor: Verbal (be) State (Quality) Minor: Connective Minor: Pronominal 3 Happening (?)	III Exp + Stat + Goal II Ent + Attr II Ent + Stat (?) Deic (Exp) (at III) Deic (Ent) (at II) Deic (Ent) (at II)
			V Purpose 4 + 3 Conn √ V Other 3 + 3⁺ ∅ √ V Other 4 + 2 Conn √ V Addition 3 + 3 Conn √ V Other 3 + 2 ∅ √ V Other (Comparative) 2 + 2 Conn √ Order-of-mention C1 → C2 → C3 √

Note: The use of an asterisk in transcription denotes overlapping speech.

PRISM–L
Summary
Name   Mr. L.   Age   55   Date of birth   ⁄

Sample no.	1						
Date	Jun. '81						
Duration	1½ mins.						
Type	Free conversa-tion						
Unanalysed	1						
Minor (p2) Types	42						
Tokens	122						
TTR	·34						
Minor:major (Tokens)	1·8						
Major (pp4-5) Types	40						
Tokens	68						
TTR	·59						
Fields used	11						
Sub-fields used	20						
Repetitions	4						

Comments

Minor Lexemes (Summary)

Unanalysed	Unintelligible *1*	Ambiguous	Symbolic Noise	Other		Totals *1*
Social	Spontaneous ooh 1 no 1 well 1		Response ah 1 well 4 thank you 1 no 4 oh 1 yes/yeah 13			
	Stereotype there you are 1		Comment you see 1 really 1			
	Proper N		Other			12 30
Relational	Pronominal 1 I 13 myself 1 2 3 it 9 you 1		Dem that 1 Art the 3 a 3 Other			
	Prepositional Loc round 2		Other of 1 Temp about 3 up to 1 Problems for 1 with 1			

	Verbal
	be 1 'm 1
	  2
	  3 is 1 's 3 been 2
	     was 2 be 3
			Other have to 2 Neg shan't 1
			might 2 not 1
			do 1 haven't 1
			'll }5 's }2
			will 've			

	Interrogative		Tags			
	Connective so 3 than 2 and 7 how 1 but 2 as though 1					
	Empty it 6 there 1 to 2		Other			Ty 30 To 92
Avoidance						Ty To

PRISM-L
Major Lexemes (Summary)

Totals Ty | 40 | .59 | | | |
To | 68 |

Page					
4	Man	Body	Health		
5	Clothing	Food			
6	Moving 3 / 5	Making/Doing 1 / 4	Happening 2 / 3	Living	
	Having	Thinking 2 / 5	Feeling		
7	Sound	Sight 2 / 3	Smell	Taste	Touch
	Language		Imagination		
8	Recreation	Occasions	Shows	Music	Art
9	Road	Rail	Air	Water	Fuel
10	Animals	Birds	Fish	Insects	
11	Flowers	Trees	Light		
	Colour	Fire	Water		
12	Building	Furniture	Tools	Containers	
13	Quantity 7 / 11	Measurement 3 / 3	Size	Shape	
	Time 4 / 5	Location 4 / 4	State 10 / 21		
14	Government	Law	Education	Religion	Business	Manufacture
15	Space	World	Minerals	Weapons	Money
	Other 2 / 4				

Moving	Come/Go go III leave I		Static		
	Sleep		Animate walk Iₒ		
	Things		Other		
Making/ Doing	General do IIIₒ		Specific		
	Type				Other
Happening	finish I ?be II				Other
Living					Other
Having	Process +		Process −		
Thinking	Process seem II think III [look I]		General		
	Type				Other
Feeling	+		−		
	Neutral		Other		

Sound	General		Quality	
	Specific		Implements	Other
Sight	Act *look* 1 *see* 11		Implements	Other
Smell	Act		Character	Other
Taste	Act		Character	Other
Touch	Act		Character	Other
Language	Speak/Listen		Read/Write	
	Act		Product	
	People		Character	
	Implements	Part		Other
Imagination	Type	People		Other

Quantity	General all I lot I other I bit II else I		Specific two I three IIII	
	Act		Other	

Measurement	Distance	Weight		Volume
	Time minute I week I year I	Heat		Other

Size	+		−	

Shape				

Time	Day		Period long II	
	Past lately I	Present now I		Future
	Frequency again I		Other	

Location	General back I here I corner I		Specific inside I	
	Part		Other	

State	Quality good (=better) III bad II•		Intensity whole I just III too I• only III very II•	
	Like + sort of I almost I		Like − otherwise I	
	Other			

Space	Entities/Events		Exploration	Other
World	Land		Water	
	Surface		Depth	
	Location	Climate		Other
Minerals	Type	Act		Other
Weapons	Type		People	Other
Money	Units		Location	
	Action	Type		Other
Other	thing III anything I			

Further Analysis

Paradigmatic Relations	Synonymy	Error
	Opposition bad/good/better inside/outside	
	Hyponymy	
	Incompatibility	
	Other	
Syntagmatic Relations		leave (re. weather (? phonological error)
Developmental Error	Overextension	
	Underextension	
	Mismatch	

PRISM–G	Name Mr. L.	Age 55	Sample Free conv. (1½ mins.)	Totals

Unanalysed

Unintelligible	Incomplete	Symbolic Noise	Ambiguous	Stereotypes	
1	2		2		5

I

Minor

Social	Proper Name	Other		+ Specifications	
26		3		2	29

C/E

Major

Elements	Activity		Entity		Deictic				Attr	Inter-rog	Other	3
	Dyn	Stat	Anim	Inanim	Anim	Inanim	Sco	Other				
							2		1			
												D
												2
		Cop										

+ Specification												
Scope							1					
Attribute												
Definiteness												
Possessive												
Quantity												S
Other							2		1			6

II

C

Elements	Act + Dyn	Exp + Stat	Poss + Stat	+ Interrog	12
		3			

	Dyn	Stat	Goal	Temp	Loc	Other
Dyn			1			1
Stat						

	Ent	Attr	Temp	Loc	Other
Ent		4			1

E

Other + Other	

24

+ Specification	Dyn	Stat	Act	Exp	Goal	Temp	Loc	Ent	Poss	Attr	Other
Scope											
Attribute											
Definiteness											
Possessive											
Quantity						1					
Other		3			1					4	

S

9

D

	Deictic							
			4	1		1	5	

11

III

Elements	+ Goal	+ Temp	+ Loc	+ Other
Act + Dyn	1	1	1	
Exp + Stat	3			
Poss + Stat				
Dyn + Goal				
Stat + Goal				
Other	Ent + Attr + Temp 1 Goal + Stat + Dyn 1			

+ Interrog

C **8**

E **24**

+ Specification	Dyn	Stat	Act	Exp	Poss	Goal	Temp	Loc	Other
Scope							2	1	
Attribute						1			
Definiteness						2		1	
Possessive									
Quantity						1	2		
Other	2	1				1	1	1	1

S **17**

	Dyn	Stat	Act	Exp	Poss	Goal	Temp	Loc	Other
Deictic	2		3			1	1		1

D **8**

IV

Elements	+ Temp	+ Loc	+ Other
Act + Dyn + Goal	2		
Exp + Stat + Goal			
Poss + Stat + Goal			
Other	Act + Dyn + Dyn + Goal 1 Act + Dyn + Stat + Goal 1		

+ Interrog

C **4**

E **16**

+ Specification	Dyn	Stat	Act	Exp	Poss	Goal	Temp	Loc	Other
Scope							1		
Attribute									
Definiteness									
Possessive									
Quantity							1		
Other	6		1						

S **9**

	Dyn	Stat	Act	Exp	Poss	Goal	Temp	Loc	Other
Deictic	5					2			

D **7**

5+ Elements		

C E

D S

Deictic		+ Specification

Totals		Means	
Major clauses (C)	27	Elements per clause (E/C)	2·5
Major elements (E)	67	Specifications per element (S/E)	·61
Specifications (S)	41	Deictics per element (D/E)	·42
Deictics (D)	28		

V

Unanalysed

Clause (A–B) Sequence

	Addition Conn	φ	Reform. Conn	φ	Contrast Conn	φ	Temporal Conn	φ	Cause Conn	φ	Location Conn	φ	Condition Conn	φ	Purpose Conn	φ	Other Conn	φ
1 + 1 ✓																		
×																		
1 + 2 ✓																		
×																		
1 + 3⁺ ✓																		
×																		
2 + 1 ✓																		1
×																		
2 + 2 ✓																	1	2
×																		
2 + 3⁺ ✓																		
×																		
3 + 1 ✓																		1
×																		
3 + 2 ✓	1						1											1
×																		
3 + 3⁺ ✓	1														1			2
×																		
4⁺ + 1 ✓																		
×																		
4⁺ + 2 ✓															1			
×																		
4⁺ + 3⁺ ✓															1			
×																		

Order-of-mention

	$C_1 \rightarrow C_2$	$C_1 \rightarrow C_2 \rightarrow C_3$	Other →	$C_2 \leftarrow C_1$	Other ←
✓	1	2			
×					

Presupposed T elements

	1 Act/Exp	Dyn/Stat	Goal	Scope	Other	2	3+	Clause
✓	1				1	2		2
×								

Idiomatic

Error

The contrast between a relatively advanced grammatical ability and an extremely restricted, 'empty' semantic ability emerges very clearly from this sample. The PRISM-L procedure shows a very narrow lexical range, with only 11 fields (20 subfields) in use. These fields cluster into two broad types, relating to pages 6 and 7 and to page 13 of the chart. The former group involves the fields Moving, Doing, Thinking, Happening and Sight, and general process lexemes (with the exception of *finish*). The latter group involves the fields Quantity, Time, Measurement (Time), Location, State and Other (*thing*), primarily for the expression of general, inspecific notions (the repeated use of *three* may be perseverative). 40 lexical types generate 68 tokens, producing a TTR of .59, which would seem to be fairly low (the nearer the TTR approaches 1.0, the less lexical repetition there is). The minor items show quite a good lexical range for the various categories represented, especially for auxiliary verbs and connectives. The Minor TTR of .34 indicates a great deal of repetition, however, and suggests that there may be automatic expression, stereotyping or other such influences affecting the speech. The overall ratio of Minor: Major is 1.8, which is very low, reflecting P's poor use of major lexemes and his full use of minor ones.

PRISM-G shows P using 27 clauses and 67 elements altogether, producing a quite advanced ratio of 2.5 elements per clause (i.e. LARSP Stage III–IV). His Stage V is also shaping up well, for such a small sample: he is able to process combinations of up to 4 elements, it seems, without error (though the lexical 'emptiness' of some of these combinations may be an underlying factor accounting for this ability). Clause elements are on the whole well specified: 41 specifications for 67 elements produces a TTR of .61—in other words, there is a 61 per cent chance of a clause element being specified (which would correlate with a fairly well developed Phrase column on the LARSP chart). On the other hand, 42 per cent of all clause elements are deictics—and it is in fact this considerable reliance on these items which makes P's speech so difficult to follow at times. He continually introduces new topics using a deictic form, which forces T to read in what he must be talking about, and causes considerable difficulties when topics are less predictable than the ones in the above sample. P's use of deictic forms, moreover, increases from about one per clause at Stage II to nearly two per clause at Stage IV—in other words, the more advanced the clause, the more the reliance on deictics, which suggests some kind of upper limit on his information-processing ability. P's weakest semantic roles seem to be Act/Exp/Ent: these have the greatest proportion of deictic exponence, and have hardly any specifications. By contrast, Goal, Temp and Loc are well specified.

In this way, a reasonably precise account of P's semantic areas of weakness can be obtained. It is difficult to make an unambiguous assessment, in view of the lack of normative data: the interpretations of TTR values, for instance, are inevitably only impressions. But it should now be possible to make some reasoned decisions concerning any structured remediation programme which it might be felt desirable to introduce. One of the first things to do would be to introduce a more specific lexical range from one of the early semantic fields, to see whether P would be able to maintain his grammatical level when faced with the need to cope with greater lexical content. Another would be to check systematically through the range of basic semantic patterns not represented in the sample, to confirm P's apparently very good comprehension skills, and to establish whether any posed particular expressive difficulties. A similar check could be made of the lexical fields, which T could continue to monitor in subsequent sessions. Semantic analysis is too much in its infancy to be able to make systematic predictions about all the avenues of remediation available. The first step, as ever, is to become aware of the complexity of the problem—the multifaceted nature of semantic difficulty, for which, it would seen, the term PRISM appears to be an apt metaphor.

Bibliographical notes

1.3 See further, D. Crystal, *Clinical linguistics* (Vienna and New York: Springer, 1981), 5ff. Further references to this book will use the abbreviation *CL*.

1.5 This theme is developed in 'Terms, time and teeth', *BJDis.Comm.* 17 (1982), 3–19.

1.6.1 For a useful discussion of the problems and principles of language testing, see S.P. Corder, *Introducing applied linguistics* (Harmondsworth: Penguin, 1973), Ch.14.

1.6.3 For a recent introduction, see J. Lyons, *Language and linguistics* (Cambridge University Press, 1981).

1.6.3(c) The point about applied linguistics is discussed further in my *Directions in applied linguistics* (London: Academic Press, 1981), Ch.1.

1.9 The clinical significance of the 'Other' category is illustrated for grammar in D. Crystal, *Working with LARSP* (London: Edward Arnold, 1979), 12–14. Further references to this book will use the abbreviation *WWL*.

1.10 For a critique of simple quantitative measures, see D. Crystal, P. Fletcher and M. Garman, *The grammatical analysis of language disability* (London: Edward Arnold, 1976), 9–11. Further references to this book will use the abbreviation *GALD*.

1.10.1 The acquisition argument is presented fully in *GALD*, 25–32; see also *WWL*, 14–15. For a review of language acquisition studies, see P. Fletcher and M. Garman (eds), *Language acquisition* (Cambridge University Press, 1979). See also A.J. Elliot, *Child language* (Cambridge University Press, 1981), esp. 33.

1.11.1 Sampling is discussed further in *GALD*, Ch.5. See also J. Miller, *Assessing language production in children* (London: Edward Arnold, 1981).

1.11.2 See *WWL*, 7–11.

2.1 As the LARSP has been expounded in detail elsewhere, the illustration and discussion in this chapter will be kept to a minimum. Further discussion of relevant points will be found in the various sections of *GALD* and *WWL*, to which appropriate references are made. See also *CL*, Ch. 4.

2.2 On sampling, see *GALD*, 86–90, *WWL*, 21–4.

2.3 On transcription, see *GALD*, 90–3, *WWL*, 24.

2.5 See further, *GALD*, 94, *WWL*, 25–33. *Stereotyped* utterances have been added to Section A in the 1981 edition of LARSP.

2.6 For discussion of the acquisitional principle, see *GALD*, 59–62, *WWL*, 14–15.

2.7 Stage I is presented in *GALD*, 63–6, *WWL*, 61–2. In the first edition of LARSP, Social Minor sentences were not subclassified, and Stereotyped sentences (now in Section A), were located at Stage I.

2.7.2 In the first edition of LARSP, an *exclamatory* sentence type was recognized; this is now located at Stage VI (see 2.14.1).

2.8 Stage II is presented in *GALD*, 67–70, *WWL*, 63–8. In the first edition of LARSP, C and O elements were not given separate lines (here and at later stages).

2.8.1 Clause elements are given a detailed explanation in R. Quirk, S. Greenbaum, G. Leech and J. Svartvik, *A grammar of contemporary English (GCE)* (London: Longman, 1972), Chs. 2, 7. See also *GALD*, Ch.3.

2.8.3 Phrase elements are described in *GCE*, 2.11, and also in Chs. 3, 4, 6, 13.

2.9 Hierarchy is discussed in *WWL*, 68–74. In the 1981 edition, transitional lines are drawn across the whole chart.

2.10 Word endings are discussed in *GALD*, 72–3, *WWL*, 84–7.

2.11 Stage III is presented in *GALD*, 70–2, *WWL*, 74–8. The distinctions between $Pron_o^p$ and Aux_o^m (in 2.11.2) were not made in the first edition of LARSP. The verb phrase is further discussed in *WWL*, 132–40. N Adj N is no longer separately specified (but logged under Other).

2.12 Stage IV is presented in *GALD*, 73–5, *WWL*, 78–84. The symbols in the Question column are more explicit versions of those used in the first edition. Tag questions are now included at this stage. Also, SVOC is now separately specified.

2.13 Stage V is presented in *GALD*, 75–7, *WWL*, 87–93. The first edition of LARSP had the Conn. column in the centre of the chart, and statement clause structure was laid out differently, but there are no substantive changes in these areas between the two editions. The distinction between Coord and Other in the Question/Command columns is novel.

2.14 Stage VI is presented in *GALD*, 77–80, *WWL*, 93–101.

2.14.2 The present chart contains a more systematic account of error types than in the first edition of LARSP.

2.15 Stage VII is presented in *GALD*, 81–3, *WWL*, 101–4.

2.16 Sections B and C are discussed in *GALD* 94–7, *WWL*, 33–55. Section D is introduced in *WWL*, 55–60, but was not on the first edition of the LARSP chart. The present edition also subclassifies Section C, and adds the category of Reduced major to Section B.

2.17 The bottom line is further illustrated in WWL, 104–5.

2.21 For other examples of this interaction, see *WWL*, Part 2.

3.1 For the theoretical background to the analysis of phonological disability see *CL*, Ch.2; also P. Grunwell, *The nature of phonological disability in children* (London: Academic Press, 1981) and D. Ingram, *Phonological disability in children* (London: Edward Arnold, 1976) and *Procedures for the phonological analysis of children's language* (Baltimore: University Park Press, 1981).

3.2 For the role of transcription in phonological analysis, see E. Carney, 'Inappropriate abstraction in speech-assessment procedures', *B J Dis.Comm.* 14 (1979), 123–35.

3.2.1 For the significance of variability, see C.A. Ferguson and C.B. Farwell, 'Words and sounds in early language acquisition', *Language* 51, 419–39; L.B. Leonard, L.E. Rowan, B. Morris and M.E. Fey, 'Intra-word phonological variability in young children', *J Ch.Lang.* 9 (1982); see also Ingram (1976, *ibid.*), Ch. 6.

3.3(a) For the characteristics of different phonological models, see *CL*, 23–34.

3.3(b) 'Progress Report: the phonetic representation of disordered speech', *B J Dis.Comm.* 15 (1980), 215–20.

3.3(c) A.C. Gimson, *An introduction to the pronunciation of English* (3rd edn, London: Edward Arnold, 1980).

3.5.1 For syllable analysis, see Gimson, *ibid.*, Ch.5; also E. Fudge, 'Syllables', *J Ling.* 5 (1969), 253–86. The respective merits of syllable-based and word-based approaches to phonological analysis are discussed in *CL*, 30–1, and Grunwell, *ibid.*

3.5.2(b) An influential discussion of syllabic division in J.D. O'Connor and J.L.M. Trim, 'Vowel, consonant and syllable—a phonological definition', *Word* 9

(1953), 103–22. Ts should beware reading in historical morphological boundaries which no longer exist, e.g. *nothing* as [nʌfɪŋ] is not [nʌ] + [fɪŋ], but [nʌ] + [f] + [ɪŋ]. Ingram (1981, *ibid.*) uses the term 'ambisyllabic' for this indeterminate category.

3.7 For regional accent differences, see A. Hughes and P. Trudgill, *English accents and dialects* (London: Edward Arnold, 1979).

3.12 The features of connected speech are classified in Gimson, *ibid.*, Ch.10.

3.16 The reasons for the missing acquisitional dimension are fully discussed in *CL*, 34–42.

3.21.1 For a brief account of these binary features, see *CL*, 26–7. A full explanation may be found in P. Ladefoged, *A course in phonetics* (New York: Harcourt, Brace, Jovanovich, 1975), Chs.11,12). For a discussion in terms of redundancy, see Carney, *ibid.*

3.21.3 For a procedure based on processes, see L.D. Shriberg and J. Kwiatkowski *Natural process analysis* (New York: Wiley, 1980), and now Ingram (1981, *ibid.*).

3.23 The task of finding monosyllabic minimal pairs in English is much facilitated by D. Rockey, *Phonetic lexicon* (London: Heyden, 1973).

4.1 See *CL*, Ch.3, esp. 58–60.

4.3 See *CL*, 62–6; also my *Prosodic systems and intonation in English* (Cambridge University Press, 1969).

4.3.3 The figures are taken from *Prosodic systems and intonation in English*.

4.4 See *CL*, 66–74.

4.5 Tone-unit disability is discussed in *CL*, 77–80.

4.5.2 The dialogue extract is taken from Exercise 20 of *WWL*, 300–1. See *WWL*, 340–1 for a grammatical analysis.

4.5.3 The importance of prosody in the analysis of 'fluent' aphasic speech is argued in *CL*, 168–73.

4.5.4 See *Prosodic systems and intonation in English*, Ch. 7, on the semantic functions of intonation.

4.6 Tone disability is discussed in *CL*, 83–7.

4.7 Tonicity disability is discussed in *CL*, 80–3.

4.9 A longer extract from this P is given in *CL*, 88–91.

5.1 The theoretical background to the notions used in this Chapter is presented in *CL*, Ch.5. See also J. Lyons, *Semantics* (Cambridge University Press, 1977), F.R. Palmer, *Semantics* (2nd edn, Cambridge University Press, 1980).

5.3(a) For lexemes, see *CL*, 137–41.

5.3(c) See further, *CL*, 135–7.

5.3(d) For example (of a specific convention), the item might be underlined, placed in brackets etc.

5.7.1 Some relevant discussion of the acquisition of semantic fields is in *CL*, 177–8. See also, A. Rescorla, 'Category development in early language', *J Ch. Lang.* 8, 225–38.

5.7.3 On the problems of semantic fields, see *CL*, 142–5, and Lyons, Palmer, *ibid.*

5.7.7 For an exposition of these paradigmatic and syntagmatic relations, see *CL*, 147–53, 153–5.

5.9.2 For examples of semantic functions, including some of the less central ones, see *CL*, 160–2; also, G. Wells, 'Learning to code experience through language', *J Ch.Lang.* 1, 243–69.

5.9.4 Deictic clinical problems are illustrated in *CL*, 119–27. See also the case-study below.

Index